Social Crisis and Mental Health

This book focuses on the paradoxical effect of social crises on mental health. When crises occur, there's an upsurge of mental suffering due to an intensification of such social insanities as violence, inequality, and insecurity. Paradoxically, there are positive consequences due to acts of kindness, cooperation, and the ability to cope and hope.

Two interconnected categories of social crises are covered in the book. These are as follows: contagions (for example, the COVID-19 pandemic, numerous outbreaks of plague and smallpox since medieval times, and the 1918 influenza pandemic); conflicts (including the Russian invasion of Ukraine, and aspects of world war such as the Holocaust, the use of nuclear bombs in the Second World War, and the climate emergency). What is also explored in the book is whether there is an amplification of everyday difficulties whereby having a 'mental health problem' has become normalised. The idea of 'mental-healthism' is introduced to explain the cultural shift towards this apparent normalisation of ordinary psychological suffering.

The book will be of interest to students, practitioners, and researchers from sociology, psychology, nursing, social work, and psychiatry, among others.

Peter Morrall is Visiting Associate Professor in Health and Sociology at the University of Leeds, UK, and a Tutor at the Centre for Lifelong Learning, University of York, UK. Morrall has worked in the mental health field and researched, written, and taught about the subject for decades.

Routledge Studies in the Sociology of Health and Illness

For more information about this series, please visit: https://www.routledge.com/
Routledge-Studies-in-the-Sociology-of-Health-and-Illness/book-series/RSSHI

Social Crisis and Mental Health

Signs of Sanity

Peter Morrall

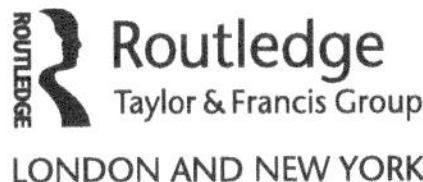

Routledge
Taylor & Francis Group

LONDON AND NEW YORK

First published 2024
by Routledge
4 Park Square, Milton Park, Abingdon, Oxon OX14 4RN

and by Routledge
605 Third Avenue, New York, NY 10158

Routledge is an imprint of the Taylor & Francis Group, an informa business

British Library Cataloguing-in-Publication Data
A catalogue record for this book is available from the British Library

ISBN: 978-1-032-12247-2 (hbk)
ISBN: 978-1-032-60652-1 (pbk)
ISBN: 978-1-003-22375-7 (ebk)

DOI: 10.4324/9781003223757

Typeset in Sabon
by codeMantra

Contents

Preface

Warning! What follows in the preface to this book is anecdotal.

In June 2022 I travelled to Tanzania, hired a motorcycle (for those who are interested, it was a Royal Enfield Himalayan), and rode from Arusha near Mount Kilimanjaro into Kenya, then Uganda, and back to Tanzania. Most of the journey involved riding through non-tourist rural areas of these countries and where I was the only non-African. I passed through hundreds of villages and towns, as well as passing by thousands of single dwellings most of which were either made wholly of mud or of brick with a corrugated metal roof. During what is now a long lifetime, I have travelled in this way (off-the-beaten-track by motorbike) to and within more than 50 countries.[1] Added to this tally are 15 or so countries using more traditional modes of transport (mostly buses, trains, and boats) to get 'off-the-beaten-track'. This journeying has taken me to six of the world's seven continents. Fellow motorcyclist Jacqui Furneaux comments about her extensive travelling:

> [A]s Einstein said, "The only source of knowledge is experience, everything else is just information" - I mused that even then you are often left with more questions than answers.[2]
>
> (Furneaux, 2021, p.82)

My wandering started in earnest in 1979 when I followed the 'hippie trail' by travelling overland from London to Srinagar in Northern India, and onward either by aeroplane or overland to other Far Eastern countries. Nearly every aspect of this 1979 journey conveyed culture shocks. But one constant shock was deep deprivation. This included a lack of basic sanitation and access to clean water and multitudes of ragged and homeless adults and children. However, there were those who were, by comparison, resource-rich. What struck me on my recent travelling is how there are still two distinct worlds. The distinction exists between and within countries and continents. The only difference is that now there are intermediate groupings, but many of these teeter on the brink of poverty rather than being *en route* to riches.

There are alternative descriptions for this distinctiveness either based on abstract and geographical separateness (for example, the West versus the rest), or stages of economic, political, and cultural development (specifically, those parts of the world that are 'developed', others that are 'developing', and failing or failed states). More recently, the global population has been split based on income (low, lower-middle, upper-middle, and high). No matter what technique and terminology is used, there is an acceptance that the boundaries of these groupings are somewhat arbitrary and amorphous, with 'shades of grey' amongst extremes. But what I observe in my journeying is that there is a persistently unambiguous and unadulterated distinct bifurcation analogous to that made by Karl Marx. It was Marx who regarded the history of humanity as essentially dissectible into two groupings based on power. Those in one group controlled all or most of the valuable resources in its respective society (for example, land, money, weaponry, personal prestige, and ideology), and wielded soft or hard power to maintain control over those resources. Those in the other group were not only deprived of control over resources but over their own lives including any awareness that this way of structuring society needn't be, and shouldn't be, tolerated.

One world is inhabited by those who are conspicuously materially, educationally, and occupationally impoverished. The other world is inhabited by those who are, in comparison, conspicuously materially, educationally, and occupationally prosperous. The ratio of the population between these two worlds has changed. But the demarcation is still stark, with any apparent intermediate groups tending to sponsor the powerful not the powerless despite the vulnerability of their structural position in society.

This divide means there is also a stark difference in both physical and psychological suffering. Morbidity and mortality rates are dissipatedly different. People in one world suffer far more from serious diseases and die much younger compared to those in the other world. While those in one world are unlikely to encounter let alone be diagnosed or offered treatment by a psychiatrist, clinical psychologist, or psychotherapist, those in the other world are susceptible to or seek professionalised stamping and succour for their psychological suffering. Social crises, such as COVID-19, homicides and suicides, and environmental emergencies, affect one world far more than the other world.

During my recent and past travelling in Africa, I have come across people who are patently in severe mental distress, dishevelled, dirty, and desolate. However, when talking with locals (I only speak a few words of Swahili, so conversations were in English accompanied by much non-verbal gesturing), a common reply to my not-very-high-quality qualitative line of questioning was that they were happy or at least not unhappy (although happiness is not necessarily equitable to mental wellness or even contentment). Society and humans are replete with paradoxes. It's complicated. Social crises add complexity and paradox. But social crises also reveal persistent characteristics of human performance often obscured by the hustle and bustle of everyday living.

In this book, I will concentrate on examining the empirical and theoretical information regarding the effects of specific and intensive social crises on mental health that I have placed under the rubrics of 'contagions' and 'conflicts' (including the COVID-19 pandemic[3] and the climate emergency[4]). However, in the background is my awareness, gained from first-hand experiences, that the most contagious and conflicted social crisis is the ongoing cultural, economic, and political impoverishment of a substantial segment of humanity. It is the catastrophe of humans living and dying in dehumanised conditions that helps feed these specific crises. The conditions in which humans exist are inexorably linked to mental health, but as already noted, this linkage is not clear-cut.

What has been patent during my perambulations are the positive-negative paradoxes in human performance: cruelty coexists with compassion, selfishness with solidarity, nonsense with sense, and resignation with resilience. But it is the positive side of the paradoxes that gives hope for a saner society, and where there are signs of a saner society there is hope for a lessening of psychological suffering.

Notes

1 After Africa that year I motorcycled from my home city of York to and back from 'Asia Minor' going through the Netherlands, Germany, Czechia, Slovakia, Hungary, Romania, Moldova, Bulgaria, Turkey, Greece, Serbia, and Austria. Towards the end of the year I motorcycled in Guatemala, El Salvador, and Honduras. The following year I rode on a motorcycle across crossed Australia (south to north).

2 This may be a misquote of Einstein for 'Learning is experience. Everything else is just information' or he may have said both phrases. The original source for either is obscure.

3 The severe acute respiratory syndrome coronavirus 2 (COVID-19/SARS-CoV-2) virus pandemic was declared over by the World Health Organisation on 5 May 2023 (WHO Europe, 2023).

4 I have tried to moderate my contribution to humanity's conflict with nature by 'off-setting' and limiting future travelling by aeroplane, walking or cycling as much as possible rather than using combustion-engine vehicles, and following a vegan diet. However, I am aware that these measures do not reconcile the arrant hypocrisy of proselytising for a saner society, on the one hand, and, on the other, indulging some of society's insanities. This is only one of my personal complex paradoxes.

References

Furneaux J (2021) (third edition) *Hit the Road, Jac! Seven Years, Twenty Countries, No Plan*. Ilkeston, UK: Shuvvy Press.

World Health Organisation Europe (2023) Coronavirus Disease (COVID-19) Pandemic – Overview. WHO Europe: Copenhagen, Denmark https://www.who.int/europe/emergencies/situations/covid-19 [accessed 8th May, 2023]

Introduction

Social crises that result from, for example, pandemics and wars furnish physical injury and fatalities and injure, possibly fatality, the organisation of a society. Social crises are also associated with psychological suffering. But a deterioration in mental health is not inexorable. Mental well-being may be sustained if not improved during a social crisis. The psychological suffering of some caused by a social crisis may contribute to the corrosion or collapse of society's systems and structures. However, social crises can have the effect of steadying the psyche of most thereby helping to steady (and potentially reorientate) society.

The conundrum of co-existing conditions of psychological suffering and psychological stability during social crises is the subject of this book. To comprehend that conundrum there are key underlying propositions. These are as follows: people have personal crises, but people and their crises subsist in societal settings therefore all crises are 'social'; the reverse can also be posited, that is, all social crises involve people and therefore are also personal; societal insanities such as violence, inequality, insecurity, selfishness, stupidity, and insecurity persist, but social crises offer people and society incidents and opportunities for change – for the better.

An individual may experience personal calamitous predicaments such as disabling, perhaps terminal, ill-health, or profound disruption to their customary lifestyle, for example, financial ruin, a contentious divorce, or the death of a loved one. Societies have crises whereby the social systems, structures, and norms of localised, national, transnational, and global human communities may be endangered, disrupted, or disintegrated, through, for example, disease, warfare, or ecocide. Personal and societal disasters are linked inexorably but while people partake in society, society is more than its people. That is, society is the dominant partner. Sociologist Emile Durkheim (1895) proposes that human society is *sui generis*, it exists above and beyond the sum of its parts. Thereby, neither human society nor the performance of humans can be understood merely by studying biological and psychological phenomena.

This book explores two genres of significant social crises that impact substantially mental health. These are as follows: (1) contagions (foremost

DOI: 10.4324/9781003223757-1

examples of which are the COVID-19 pandemic, and outbreaks of plague, smallpox, and influenza); (2) conflicts (focusing on aspects of world war, the invasion of Ukraine by Russia in 2022, and humanity's assault on nature that has resulted in the collapse of ecosystems and contraction in biodiversity). There are, of course, other sets of social crises that impact mental health apart from these two. Mental health can be soiled, sustained, or strengthened by any social crisis. Contagion and conflicts have been chosen because they not only envelop multiple incidents of social crises but may have relevance to those not included. Moreover, they cover a range of contemporary and historical social issues apart from crises, all of which matter to mental health. The question of whether there is a crisis in mental health will also be raised, and whether today's world can be characterised as continually in a social crisis.

Ideas and Aims

The idea for this book is to follow up on my previous book titled *Insane Society: A Sociology of Mental Health* (Morrall, 2020). In that book, the relationship between society's insanities and mental health/disorder is the focus. Five foremost insanities were identified: inequality, violence, selfishness, insecurity, and stupidity. Individually, they are the source of serious psychological suffering. Collectively, I argued, these insanities source the sweeping insanity of contemporary life.

The emphasis in this book will be on the relationship between society's sanities and mental health. To understand this relationship, a wide range of data and ideas from the natural, medical, and social sciences will support the application of the sociological imagination.

Overall, I utilise the imaginative thinking of sociologist C Wright Mills (1959). Specific ideas from, for example, the works of social psychologist, psychoanalyst, philosopher, humanist, and sociologist, Erich Fromm (1955; 1964; 1973) are inherently involved in the task of exposing societal insanities as well as providing an impulse to go beyond intellectualism by advocating activism directed towards making society saner. What such thinkers have in common is an acceptance of a dynamic and reflexive interrelationship between human performance (individual cognition, conduct, and feelings) and society (its structures, institutions, and systems). Self and society are irrevocably linked. An individual's psychological and biological make-up and societal cultural and institutional configurations are entwined.

For Mills 'private troubles' are 'public issues' and vice versa. Nature and nurture cannot be wholly disentangled, although some private troubles (for example, inherited genetic diseases: World Health Organisation, 2020) and some public issues (for example, gun crime, bad food, carbon emissions: Dowding, 2020a; 2020b) are mainly one or the other. Personal madness and societal insanity is a prime example of bio-psycho-social inseparability (Morrall, 2020; Rose, 2019; Rose and Abi-Rached, 2013). Fromm blames the cultural craziness of capitalism, totalitarian communism, and fascism for much psychological suffering. What Fromm also contributes to my way of thinking is 'positivity'. Fromm not only contributes to the identification of past and present insanities but presents a scenario for a saner society. Sociology should not just be about thought but a discipline that is secured to social responsibility to help attain that society.

In concluding my book *Insane Society: A Sociology of Mental Health* (Morrall, 2020), I suggested a revolutionary and revelatory idea, a 'Fourth Way' was necessary to show the world a saner way of living than capitalism, communism, or communitarianism have been able to deliver. But I intonated that such a new politically pragmatic idea was more likely to be forthcoming when one or more catastrophic societal insanity was imminent or transpiring. That was March 2020, just as COVID-19 was about to be recognised as a biological and societal calamity, and one with major implications for mental health (Fox and Monahan, 2020). This book is not intended to furnish fully a Fourth Way, solely solve society's insanities, nor mend most of madness. But it is intended to help to head in those directions.

The aims of this book are therefore:

1 To reaffirm the connections between societal contexts and mental health while not dismissing the role played by biological and psychological factors.
2 To explore the societal and psychological complexities and paradoxes that occur during social crises, including the co-existence of a 'mental health crisis' and a crisis of 'mental-healthism'.
3 To emphasise existing signs of societal sanities sanity and give a route to a saner society.

Complexity and Paradox

Society and humans are complicated (Goldacre, 2014; Morrall, 2020). This complexity comprises a concoction of contradictions. But the relationships between societal sanities, insanities, and mental health are consistently complicated, persistently paradoxical, and commonly concealed.

Contagions and conflicts comprise the complexity and contradiction of calamity and consolation. For Ian Goldin, a scholar of globalisation and technological and economic development, this paradox has the potential to improve humanity's lot:

> Every crisis creates an opportunity, and it behoves us to explore the silver linings.
>
> (Goldin, 2021, p.246)

Despite the undoubtedly damaging and deadly impacts of disasters, not all the effects on people and their communities from, for example, wars and plagues are inevitably pathological. The effects on the mental makeup of some of those caught in crises may be the reverse of what might be expected and what is commonly reported in the academic and clinical literature. Sociologist Charles Fritz (1996) argues that there is a need to balance the pessimistic view of social crises by identifying and validating their psychological silver linings, and fathoming why disasters produce mentally healthy conditions.

Pandemics, wars, and ecocides exemplify the societal insanities of violence, inequality, selfishness insecurity, and stupidity. They also reveal the societal sanities of kindness, cooperation, solidarity, coping, and hoping. Social insanities, social sanities, psychological suffering, and psychological stability are inexorably interrelated. However, unlike societal insanities, the benefits of societal sanities for mental health may not be manifest.

Evidence of mental distress during social crises is plentiful and patent from contemporary times but scarce or concealed regarding psychological positive payoffs. There is much less available data other than anecdotes regarding, for example, medieval pestilences (al-be-it that some were recorded contemporaneously and therefore may have a higher validity value). Judicious inferences can be made about earlier events based on what has been learned from later events. That is, comprehending how armed combat sourced severe and persistent anxiety in some soldiers during a world war is a suitable starting point for speculation that medieval battles may have had similar psychological consequences. This is not to ignore philosopher Michel Foucault's (1969) notification that the past cannot easily, if ever, be comprehended from the position of the present.[1] The 'archaeology of knowledge' (Foucault's term for his analytical method) about human performance may not reveal ultimate truths, but studying diligently all the available ideas and evidence can provide more valid understandings.

Contagions such as COVID-19 and conflicts that spread across the globe in the form of violence or the violation of the physical environment are colossal social crises and therefore are distinguishable from other calamities and from the commotion in customary life. Contagions and conflicts are also bonded. They are inseparably entwined and signify an overall crisis in human society. But, while there are no excuses for complacency about the state of the world, there is some basis for sanguinity.

The COVID-19 pandemic, the 2022 invasion of Ukraine by Russia, and the ongoing climate emergency symbolise the general insaneness of (global) society, and they have cultivated specific insanities. Societal norms during the COVID-19 pandemic altered dramatically. Mostly the alterations in how global society operates during any social crisis are conveyed as negative. There is some academic evidence and much media assertion that COVID-19 has also altered psychological states dramatically. As with the operation of society's institutions and infrastructure, most of the effects on mental health are reported as harmful. From the invasion of Ukraine, there is graphic video documentation showing the wreckage of homes, schools, and hospitals through bombing, and palpable personal testimony of psychological suffering caused by beatings, rape, and killings (Bryant *et al.*, 2022; Human Rights Watch, 2023). This conflict is unique due to the vast coverage supplied by social media and regular media together with the attention paid to many of the events as they happen or to their aftermaths because it is taking place in Europe. As the climate emergency worsens and affects Western countries more and more, it is likely that similar coverage and attention will be forthcoming. But these social crises, along with many others, also serve well for the exploration of society's sanities. No matter the dreadfulness and density of the insanities, there are some reasons to be cheerful, and if not cheerful then more doubtful in accepting humanity and its society is doomed.

Extensive claims of a secondary social crisis, a crisis in mental health, also invites doubtfulness. Rather than a legitimate crisis in mental health (or more accurately a crisis of psychological suffering) what might be happening is a process I have termed 'mental-healthism'. That is, although psychological suffering is a personal trouble for a sizeable sum of people, the description of 'crisis' is unwarranted. Most people most of the time are mostly not mentally unwell. Psychological suffering may be part of the human condition, but so is psychological steadfastness. On its journey from hominoid to Homo sapiens, from cave dwellings to global society, and notwithstanding human capacity for creating societal insanities, the human psyche has become remarkably robust.

Declarations of a crisis generate not only unwarranted political and public panic but also warranted personal and societal properties. Atypical times can give rise to interpersonal connectivity and sensitivity when the culture of global society is typically ridden with individualism, narcissism, greediness, and brutalities. Duplicity and claptrap may become challenged by a resurgence in the value of personal integrity and the re-establishment of scientific rigour. The becalming of the environment during the COVID-19 pandemic 'lockdowns' moderated global warming and pollution, as well as personal perturbation. This contagion gave justification for politicians to curtail human rights in many countries, but there was an increase across the globe in the politicisation of personal empowerment (Bringel and Pleyers, 2022). Examples of constructive contemporaneous occurrences and corollaries of the invasion of Ukraine by Russia and the climate emergency may be less apparent than those of the COVID pandemic. Juxtaposed with death and destruction, both have very apparent negative effects on the solidity of the psyche. But these negative effects are not necessarily as widespread as is often they are purported to be in the public consciousness, and clinical and academic literature.

Whether there is a crisis in mental health or mental-healthism is rife, there are significant signs of a saner society and a boost to the solidity of the psyche. During the COVID-19 pandemic, these signs of sanity included the following: increased levels of social solidarity, charitableness, volunteering; compassion, helpfulness, mutual aid, and a sense of 'community spirit'; unprecedented support for health/medical workers, carers, emergency personnel, and other 'essential' workers; succumbing to serenity because of the becalming of traffic and closure of 'off-line' businesses; less business also meant less environmental pollution; parents and children sharing more 'quality time'; increased – if enforced – leisure time; opportunities for campaigning about, for example, ecological issues (Alberti, 2020; Kuebler, 2020; Nelson, 2020; Sitrin and Semrar, 2020; Stansfield *et al.*, 2020). Because of these personal and public progressions, there may also be a raising of the collective consciousness and conscience about how life could and should be lived differently (Conniff, 2020). There were, however, huge variations geographically and demographically within and between countries and regions as well as temporally in how the negative and positive consequences of the COVID-19 pandemic have been reified, rectified, or refuted (Williams, 2021).

The COVID pandemic shows the dynamic and reflexive linkage between the somatic, psychological, and societal. Most disasters, including the widespread dissemination of disease, are intrinsically connected with other overarching crises. Global warming and the diminution of biological diversity are the uppermost catastrophes (Ripple *et al.*, 2019; United Nations, 2020b). The General Secretary of the United Nations warns:

> [O]ur planet is broken.
>
> (Guterres, 2020, p.2)

The climate crisis and biodiversity deficiency, which are linkable directly with societal factors such as deforestation, global transport and tourism, industrial farming, and meat-consumption, are predicted to cause further and worse pandemics (Bernstein, 2020; Kuebler, 2020; Mair, 2020; Politico, 2020; Snowden, 2020; Vaughn, 2019). More pandemics and violence are likely to furnish further mental-health disasters and/or mentalhealthism. The lessons learned from such disasters, as with other all societal insanities, must not mean concentrating only on microbiology and associated technologies, regulating inter-personal contact and cleanliness, and pharmaceuticals. Global social systems, structures, and systems need renovating or replacing.

As with past disasters, whether human-made or 'natural', the profound jolt to human life and societal systems resulting from the present pandemic means the future is uncertain (Dunbar *et al.*, 2020; Mair, 2020). However, social theorist Naomi Klein (2020) argues the way individuals and society have changed for the better because of COVID needs to be captured and exploited. For Klein, these changes put humanity in a better position to deal with the standing of serious societal insanities such as the climate crisis, racism, and inequality. Societal insanities of every hue affect access to and activation of societal sanities, therefore they need to be tackled to allow the benefits of living in saner society to be distributed equally.

Historian Rutger Bregman postulates that no matter how disastrous the situation in which people find themselves or create for themselves, human goodness mostly prevails:

[M]ost people, deep down, are pretty decent.

(Bregman, 2020, p.2)

What is not yet established is how widespread and effective human and societal decency has been during the disaster of COVID-19 or will be from the invasion of Ukraine by Russia and the climate emergency, and whether this can help craft a saner society for typical times.

Terms and Topics

There are many synonyms in the relevant academic and clinical literature for what I am referring to as a 'crisis'. The most common of these are 'disaster', 'catastrophe', and 'calamity'. I will use these terms interchangeably with that of crisis. However, the expression 'social crisis' will be maintained consistently when referring to the effects on society (and its inhabitants) caused by all manner of disasters, catastrophes, and calamities. Another necessary nomenclatural clarification relates to 'natural disaster' and 'human-made disaster'. These are often considered as separate entities in the literature based on causation (nature versus humans). The argument will be made, however, that in some cases this is a false dichotomy because human activity impinges directly or indirectly on the workings of nature, the prime and devastating example of which is the climate emergency.

To date, the definition of 'social crisis' is far from definitive. Many of the attempts at definition merely refer to types of crises and how they affect society. Some definitions are guilty of intermingling teleology with tautology (by linking causes of social crises to their consequences and referring to 'social crises' as 'disasters' or *vice versa)* rather than offering a viable explanation. For example:

Social crisis refers to incidents arising from…disasters which endanger normal social order and public security causing dysfunction in the social functioning mechanism…. Not only do disasters result in casualties and the destruction of facilities, they also have a significant impact on the society and may even cause social crises.

(Xu *et al.*, 2016, p.46)

Others do attempt to go beyond description by concocting concepts intended to clarify but may confound, or only bestow partial comprehension. Sociologist Jeffrey Alexander (2019), for example, offers 'societalization' as a new theory to explain social crises. Jeffrey Alexander's theory is that social crises are triggered by how 'social strains' are interpreted rather than by actual events. When public expectations of leadership, justice, morality, and stability if not survival are perceived as being undermined then, according to Jeffrey Alexander, a 'war of the spheres' ensues. This war may be between the stances staged by society's elites (for example, those formally responsible for governance, commerce, the military, and morality) and the discernments of the disadvantaged (the poor, the exploited, the punished, and the disillusioned). In some circumstances the war shifts from internalised antagonism words to externalised violence.

Apart from the linguistic intelligence of the term, the theory of 'societalization' does not offer exhaustive enlightenment on a myriad of social crises including those that can be described as 'moral panics' to panics about plagues. Nor does it expound precisely on how strains become crises. Hence, 'societalization' may be an interesting idea regarding description but is not an explanation.

'Crisis', according to sociologist Robert Holton (1987), has become an over-used and indistinct rhetorical metaphor. The separation of normalness from crises has, posits Holton, become blurred and confused. Crises in public, political, and media discourses are reported so regularly that there is never not a crisis somewhere. Every political, economic, or cultural setback is disastrous, calamitous, a catastrophe, a watershed, or an emergency. But Holton is adamant that society (he is specifically referring to the West) is not in total crisis.

However, the opening speech at the G20 summit of world leaders held in Bali in October 2022, Indonesia's President Joko Widodo commented on the state of the world. He warned that:

> Crisis after crisis still haunts the world.
>
> (Widodo quoted in Karmini, 2022)

The charity International Rescue Committee lists scores of crises. Related to contagion, conflict, and the climate during 2021–2022 these include: famine (for example, Yemen, Nigeria, Kenya, and the Democratic Republic of Congo); drought (Sudan); deforestation (for example, Brazil); internal social unrest (for example, Sudan, Argentina, Iran, Russia, Mali, and Myanmar); infestation (for example, locust swarms in South Sudan and Ethiopia); internal displacement (Burkina Faso); economic inflation, recession, or collapse (for example, the UK, Turkey, Lebanon, Afghanistan, and Syria); escalating criminality (for example, Honduras).

Such a compendium of crises for the International Rescue Committee points to a systemic failure for tens of millions of people.

> Each day that the system for guaranteeing peace and prosperity fails, human suffering grows. Business as usual is not good enough. For the people the IRC serves, now is the time for a total system upgrade.
>
> (International Rescue Committee, 2022, p.3)

It is difficult to imagine how this failed system and the need for its upgrade do not imply that the whole of society is not failing and that the whole of society, therefore, needs upgrading.

At the time of writing this book, 2023, social crises seem pervasive and intractable. This period is noticeable in the number of serious social crises it is experiencing. Diseases, blood-shedding, and/or environmental calamities have occurred in the Democratic Republic of Congo, Myanmar, Sudan, Syria, Somalia, South Sudan, Nigeria, Yemen, Ethiopia, and Afghanistan (International Rescue Committee, 2022). In 2007/2008, there was an unprecedented global financial which nearly caused the international banking system to collapse, and that would have undermined if not annihilated global trade with devastating social and psychological consequences. Since then, further financial crises have occurred, although more localised. In 2022 specific monetary mishaps affected, for example, Lebanon, Sri Lanka, Cape Verde, Ecuador, Argentina, Egypt, Zimbabwe, and Pakistan. Moreover, alongside and related to the ongoing COVID-19 pandemic, the disastrous invasion of Ukraine by Russia, an 'economic emergency' occurred in Europe including the UK. Covering most of the front page of the British newspaper The Daily Mirror on 27 August 2022 was this headline tagged as 'message to our leaders':

> Our whole country is facing an energy bills catastrophe. For heaven's sake do something.

In the year 2023, speakers at a conference held by the United Nations predicted a 'grim picture' of more suffering, deaths, mass migration, and violence, due to what they identified as a 'global water crisis' unless appropriate financing, infrastructure, and policies were adopted urgently (United Nations Water Conference, 2023). By 2023, not only had the Russian and Ukraine economies become undermined by the deliberate devastation of Ukraine's infrastructure and the trading restrictions placed on Russia, but the world economy had been hit by 'doom and gloom' (Low and Millard, 2023). But the worst global financial disaster to date happened years before the President of the Russian Federation ordered the invasion of its neighbour.

The Department of Economic and Social Affairs of the United Nations (UNDESA, 2011) reports on what it refers to as the 'global social crisis' triggered by the near collapse of the world's core financial system in 2007 and 2008. Financial instability had negative consequences for billions of people, thousands of communities, and a myriad of national and global systems of production and distribution. There was a rise in levels of poverty, hunger, unemployment, crime, gender-based violence, substance abuse, and mental illness, including depression and suicide. Previous economic failures such as the Great Depression of the late 1920s and throughout the 1930s, the 1997 financial slumps in Thailand, South Korea, Indonesia, Hong Kong, Laos, Malaysia, and the Philippines, and, although to a lesser extent, in Brunei, mainland China, Singapore, Taiwan, and Vietnam, are associated with increases in morbidity, including psychological suffering, and mortality, including suicide (UNDESA, 2011).

Terms and Title

A word about terminology is necessary. In previous publications, I have adopted the term 'madness' when referring to psychological suffering that may be diagnosed as mental disorder. The term 'madness' has been in Western countries and still is used in the few remaining traditional cultures to describe behaviours, thoughts, or emotions considered by the populace and/or the powerful as unacceptable, odd, or dangerous. Madness has traditionally been associated with any number of gods, the devil, rather than primarily with personal biological and psychological pathology (Hirst and Woolley, 1982; Porter, 1987). Madness in this sense is a pre-medicalisation or non-medicalised signing of irregular and undesirable acts, beliefs, and feelings. The sociologist Andrew Scull (2015) notes that using the term madness attracts criticism that it is politically incorrect. For Scull and me, however, it remains a common-sense designation and one which is decoupled from medicalisation. When referring to a formal medical diagnosis, I will adopt the relevant psychiatric term rubric of mental disorder (or mental illness) or the name of the specific disorder. But this should not be taken as an acceptance by me of medical definitional or conceptual legitimacy.

My use of the expression 'psychological suffering' refers to a state of mind that an individual experiences in one way or another as negative. Some forms of psychological suffering (such as severe fearfulness or sadness, or feelings of persecution) could become classified as 'madness' in the sociological sense or medicalised as 'mental disorder'). Not all forms of psychological suffering, however, are unwanted or unfavourable. 'Psychological stability' (or the synonyms of steadfastness, sturdiness, and solidity) denotes a mental state characterised by an ability to cope and be composed, and possibly feel contentment. The term 'psychological progression' (or 'psychological prosperity') is used to describe how a stable mental state may advance beyond just coping and composure whereby the individual wants to and does make improvements to her/his way of thinking, behaving, and/or emotional experiences. Psychological suffering and psychological stability are interlinked and are always both private and public. They have both personal and societal causes, contexts, and consequences. There is also the interlinking of personal hardiness and malleability with sustainability and adaptability, both affected by and affecting each other.

'Signs of Sanity' is the title of a book published in 1922 by Stewart Patton. Patton, a medical practitioner, neurobiologist, and 'mental hygienist', offers this clear definition of the difference between sanity and insanity:

> Sanity is a successful, and insanity and unsuccessful, attempt to adjust life to reality.
>
> (Patton, 1922, p.2)

For Patton, the functioning of every organism is the consequence of both heredity and the environment. The same is true, argues Patton, for sane and insane human performance. It follows that Patton regards mind and body as intimately connected. A sound mind and a sound body (especially but not exclusively the brain) are interdependent. He is making the case that sanity and insanity can only be understood through the understanding of the psychological and biological make-up of humans along with their social and physical contexts. On the downside of his otherwise morally and intellectually shrewd thinking, Patton supported eugenics, and in 1919 he served as president of the USA Eugenics Research Association (Rogers, 1965).

On another issue relating to the style of writing adopted in the book, there will be limited use of abbreviations. Although this means repeating sometimes long-winded designations, it will help avoid confusion or the reader having to flip back and forth to find the earlier full references. For example, the Intergovernmental Panel on Climate Change will always be written in full and not replaced by 'IPCC' unless one or more references are made to that agency in close succession within the text.

Chapters and Repetition

There are six chapters, including the Introduction and Conclusion. Chapter 1 contains descriptions of social crises created by contagions and conflicts. Examples of contagion covered in the chapter are the COVID-19 pandemic, plagues, smallpox, and influenzas (as well as tuberculosis and HIV/AIDS). Specific aspects of world war conflicts will be covered (notably the Holocaust and the dropping of atomic bombs on Japan during the Second World War), the invasion of Ukraine by Russia, and the ongoing climate and biodiversity emergency. In Chapter 2 there is an assessment of the validity of describing mental health as being in 'crisis', and in Chapter 3 there is the presentation of 'mental-healthism' as a concept that describes levels of psychological suffering to contrast with the notion of a crisis. Chapter 4 explores the contradictory consequences of catastrophe that are indicative of psychological stability rather than psychological suffering. These 'signs of sanity' are kindness, co-operation, solidarity, coping, and hoping.

Although there is a specific topic claimed for each chapter, it has proven to be problematic to keep these separate because they interrelate. This leads to some repetition. There is also a repetition of the themes of complexity and paradox because of these interrelations, it is also due to how life and the universe are not consistently and comprehensively understood.

More Good than Bad

Notwithstanding the terrible cruelties, the destruction of physical environments, collapsing of communities, the pervasiveness of mendacity and stupidity, and the apparent ubiquity of despair and disempowerment, people do good and sensible things as do some social institutions, and personal and societal goodness and sense is good and sensible for mental health. Galvanising the personal, interpersonal, and communal positives from a social crisis can help make society less insane and psychological suffering subside. The signs of sanity seen in social crises may not solve all of society's insanities nor be the solution to all psychological suffering. But they do offer hope for a saner way of living and being.

Signs of sanity are not just the celebrated and superlative deeds of magnanimity, philanthropy, altruism, unanimity, and sensibleness. There are the multitudinous, mundane, and minuscule endeavours that seed those venerated successes. These usually inconspicuous acts fertilise the foundations that could furnish a saner society and thereby secure psychological stability if not psychological progress.

Note

1 Incomprehensively, despite Foucault claiming history is incomprehensibly, he applies his idiosyncratic genealogical schema of 'knowledge archaeology' to do just that (Foucault, 1969).

References

Alberti F (2020) Coronavirus Is Revitalising the Concept of Community for the 21st Century. The Conversation, 29th April. https://theconversation.com/coronavirus-is-revitalising-the-concept-of-community-for-the-21st-century-135750 [accessed 7th May, 2020]

Bregman R (2020) *Human Kind: A Hopeful History*. London: Bloomsbury.

Bernstein A (2020) Coronavirus, Climate Change, and the Environment: A Conversation on COVID-19 with Dr. Aaron Bernstein, Director of Harvard Chan C-CHANGE Center for Climate, Health, and the Global Environment at the Harvard T.H. Chan School of Public Health. Harvard University.

Bringel B and Pleyers G (2022) (editors) *Social Movements and Politics During COVID-19: Crisis, Solidarity and Change in a Global Pandemic*. Bristol: Bristol University Press.

Bryant R, Schnurr P and Pedlar D (2022) Addressing the Mental Health Needs of Civilian Combatants in Ukraine. *The Lancet Psychiatry*, 9(5), pp.346–347.

Conniff R (2020) How Devastating Pandemics Change Us. *National Geographic Magazine*, 14th July.

Dowding K (2020a) Governments Set the Rules – So They Shouldn't Blame Us for Not Behaving Better. The Conversation, 15th September. https://theconversation.com/governments-set-the-rules-so-they-shouldnt-blame-us-for-not-behaving-better-146031 [accessed 1th September, 2020]

Dowding K (2020b) *It's the Government, Stupid: How Governments Blame Citizens for Their Own Policies*. Bristol: Bristol University Press.

Dunbar R, Zebrowski C and Olsson P (2020) Is Humanity Doomed Because We Can't Plan for the Long Term? Three Experts Discuss. The Conversation, 5th August. https://theconversation.com/is-humanity-doomed-because-we-cant-plan-for-the-long-term-three-experts-discuss-137943 [accessed 7th August, 2020]

Fox H and Monahan E (2020) *Impact On Mental Health [Well-Being, Loneliness, Depression And Anxiety]: Coronavirus (COVID-19) Review: Data and Analysis*, March to October 2020. London: Office of National Statistics [UK]. https://static.ons.gov.uk/files/covid-19-review--impact-on-mental-health.pdf. [accessed 1st December, 2002]

Foucault M (1969) *L'archéologie du Savoir*. Paris: Gallimard [Translated as The Archaeology of Knowledge, Allan Sheridan (translator), New York: Harper and Row, 1972].

Fromm E (1964) *The Heart of Man: Its Genius for Good and Evil*. New York: Harper & Row.

Fromm E. (1973) *The Anatomy of Human Destructiveness*. New York: Holt, Rinehart & Winston.

Goldacre B (2014) *I Think You'll Find It's a bit More Complicated Than That*. London: Fourth Estate.

Goldin I (2021) *Rescue: From Global Crisis to a Better World*. London: Spectre.

Guterres A (2020) *State of the Planet*. New York: United Nations. https://www.un.org/sites/un2.un.org/files/sgspeech-the-state-of-planet.pdf [accessed 2nd December, 2020]

Hirst P and Woolley P (1982) *Social Relations and Human Attributes*. London: Tavistock.

Holton R (1987) The Idea of Crisis in Modern Society. *British Journal of Sociology*, 38(4), pp. 502–520.

https://www.nationalgeographic.com/magazine/2020/08/how-devastating-pandemics-change-us-feature/ [accessed 8th October, 2020]

https://www.sciencedirect.com/science/article/pii/S2590198220301299 [accessed 13th December, 2020]

https://www.theguardian.com/society/2020/oct/17/uk-sleepwalking-to-mental-health-crisis-as-pandemic-takes-its-toll [accessed 20th October, 2020]

Human Rights Watch (2023) *World Report 2023*. New York: Human Rights Watch.

Klein N (2020) 'We must not return to the pre-Covid status quo, only worse'. Quoted by Viner K, [interview]. The Guardian, 13th July.

Kuebler M (2020) Legal Tactics Environmentalists Are Using to Fight Climate Change. Deutsche Welle [Deutschland], 16th November, 2020. https://www.dw.com/en/5-legal-tactics-environmentalists-are-using-to-fight-climate-change/a-55593003 [accessed 19th November, 2020]

Mair S (2020) What Will the World Be Like After Coronavirus? Four Possible Futures. The Conversation, 30th March. https://theconversation.com/what-will-the-world-be-like-after-coronavirus-four-possible-futures-134085 [accessed 12th June, 2020]

Morrall P (2020) *Insane Society: A Sociology of Mental Health*. Abingdon: Routledge.

Nelson B (2020). The Positive Effects of Covid-19. *British Medical Journal*, 369, m1785. https://www.bmj.com/content/369/bmj.m1785 [accessed 12th June, 2020]

Patton S (1922) *Signs of Sanity*. New York: Charles Scribner's Sons.

Politico (2020) Coronavirus Will Change the World Permanently: Here's How. *Politico Magazine*, 19th March. https://www.politico.com/news/magazine/2020/03/19/coronavirus-effect-economy-life-society-analysis-covid-135579. [accessed 12th June, 2020]

Porter R (1987) *A Social History of Madness: Stories of the Insane*. London: Weidenfeld & Nicolson.

Ripple W, Wolf C, Newsome T, Barnard P and Moomaw WR (2019) World Scientists' Warning of a Climate Emergency. *BioScience*, 70(1), pp.8–12. [Corrigendum, BioScience, 2020, 70(1), p.100]

Rogers F (1965) Stewart Paton (1865–1942): Mental Hygienist. *American Journal of Public Health Nations Health*, 55(5), pp.654–656.

Rose N (2019) *Our Psychiatric Future: The Politics of Mental Health*. Cambridge: Polity.

Rose N and Abi-Rached J (2013) *Neuro: The New Brain Sciences and the Management of the Mind*. Princeton, NJ: Princeton University Press.

Scull A (2015) *Madness in Civilisation: From the Bible to Freud, from the Madhouse to Modern Medicine*. London: Thames & Hudson.

Sitrin M and *Colectiva Semrara* (2020) (editors) *Pandemic Solidarity: Mutual Aid During the Covid-19 Crisi*. London: Pluto.

Snowden F (2020) (edition with Covid-19 preface) *Epidemics and Society: From the Black Death to the Present*. New Haven, CT: Yale University Press.

Stansfield J, Mapplethorpe T and South J (2020) The Community Response to Coronavirus (COVID-19) Public Health England (Blog), 1st June 2020. The Community Response to Coronavirus (COVID-19) – Public Health Matters (blog.gov.uk) [accessed 27th November, 2020]

United Nations (2020b) *Biodiversity in Grave Danger: What Can Be Done in 2020?* New York: United Nations. https://www.unenvironment.org/news-and-stories/story/biodiversity-grave-danger-what-can-be-done-2020 [accessed 4th October, 2020]

Vaughn A (2019) How Deadly Disease Outbreaks Could Worsen as the Climate Changes. New Scientist, 3253, 15th October. https://www.newscientist.com/article/2219981-how-deadly-disease-outbreaks-could-worsen-as-the-climate-changes/ [accessed 14th October, 2020]

World Health Organisation (2020) Human Genomics in Global Health: Genes and Human Diseases. Geneva. https://www.who.int/genomics/public/geneticdiseases/en/index2.html [accessed 29th Sepetember, 2020]

1   Contagions and Conflicts

In this chapter, the social crises resulting from life-threatening and life-taking infectious diseases and armed hostilities are explored. References are made to how contagions and conflicts connect to mental health, but this is explored more fully in the next chapter.

The specific focus of this chapter is on the contagions of plague, smallpox, influenza, and COVID-19, and the conflicts of Russia's invasion of Ukraine, world war (namely the Holocaust and nuclear accidents and bombings), and the confrontation between humanity and nature that has created the climate emergency. Contagions and conflicts, however, are linked. For example, contagions are the physiological pathological outcome of humanity's conflict with nature, and they can have psychological pathological effects. Humanity is also in conflict with animals. It is unlikely any animal wants to be treated badly let alone eaten by humans. Humanity and animals are also frequently conflicted by contagions, passing on to each other dangerous diseases.

First in this chapter, however, are 'scene-setting' discussions on zoonosis and disasters.

Zoonosis

All contagions have societal causes and consequences and are therefore not only medical disorders but social disorders. Human exploitation of other life forms and the increasing overlapping of human and animal living (and dying) conditions can be construed as a socially created contagious conflict.

David Quammen is the author of fiction and non-fiction books. An example of the latter is 'Spillover: Animal Infections and the Next Human Pandemic'. Quammen uses the term 'spillover' to describe the moment when a pathogen passes from one host species to another species that until then becomes a new host. Animal diseases and human diseases are interlinked. Zoonotic diseases kill humans in their millions (after all, humans are animals). The reverse also happens. Anthroponosis is the term for the transmission of human pathogens to animals, and other primates are especially vulnerable.

There is a multitude of known zoonotic diseases, many of which are dangerous if not deadly. Quammen provides examples, including bubonic

DOI: 10.4324/9781003223757-2

plague, influenzas, smallpox, AIDS/HIV, SARS, Ebola, monkeypox, bovine tuberculosis, Lyme disease, West Nile fever, Marburg virus disease, rabies, anthrax, Lassa fever, Rift Valley fever, Nipah encephalitis, and bovine spongiform encephalopathy (Mad Cow disease). Although controversial certain types of malaria, for example, *Plasmodium knowlesi* are now considered zoonotic. The controversy is about whether malaria is truly a zoonotic disease when there is an intermediary 'vector' (the mosquito) required before it is transferred into the human bloodstream (van de Straat *et al.*, 2022).

There are six types of pathogens that cause most of the zoonotic diseases. These are viruses, bacteria, protists (previously named protozoans), prions, and worms. The settings that allow zoonotic diseases to easily infect humans are the disintegration of ecosystems (through, for example, logging, slash-and-burn agriculture, hunting for 'bushmeat', pasture grazing for cattle, mineral extraction, urban sprawl, chemical pollution of land and sea, and intensive fishing), global trade and transport, and conflict.

Human exploitation of and cruelty towards animals are also key to the spread of zoonotic diseases (Quammen, 2012). In China and other Asian countries wildlife and 'wet' and seafood markets supply multiple species of live animals. They may be sold alive or slaughtered at the market and placed near live animals, possibly packed into small open wire cages one on top of another. Examples of animals in these markets include chickens, fish, shellfish, snakes, beavers, badgers, bats, ducks, geese, pheasants, magpies, cormorants, lizards, porcupines, young crocodiles, hares, and civets. Animal waste and the pathogens it contains contaminates other produce and is passed from one animal to another and one species to another including humans (Maron, 2020). Thomas Lovejoy (2021) is an ecologist. He coined the first term 'biological diversity'. For Lovejoy the COVID-19 pandemic is assuredly the consequence of persistent and excessive intrusion by humans into nature and the vast illegal wildlife trade, and, in particular, the wildlife markets, the wet markets, of South Asia, and the bush meat markets of Africa. Wet markets are traditional markets selling live animals (farmed and wild) as well as fresh fruit, vegetables, and fish, often in unhygienic conditions. They are found all over Africa and Asia, providing sustenance for hundreds of millions of people.

> It is very clear that human disruption/destruction of nature (in a negative synergy with wildlife trade and markets) constitute a recipe for enhanced probability of spillover. That is multiplied by massive populations of domesticated animals and the size of the human population. …
>
> (Lovejoy, 2021)

Quammen is scathing about the animals being farmed and mistreated. He points out the dangers to the health of animals and humans and the concomitant abuse of non-human creatures involved in the massive increase in livestock for human consumption. The desire of human consumers to be provided with meat is increasing exponentially as the global population grows. Moreover, the circumstances for animals *en route* to being consumed have become worse.

Huge factory-like facilities corral thousands of cattle, pigs, chickens, ducks, sheep, and goats. This allows the transference of disease from visiting animals (for example, bats and rats) and then on to humans, and aids the mutation of pathogens thereby making existence more sustainable and potentially far more threatening to their hosts and humans. To control this otherwise inevitable proliferation of disease, prophylactic doses of antibiotics are used on the animals, and along with other drugs used to fatten the animal; this has the added benefit for the farmer of delivering higher profits. The overuse of antibiotics in human healthcare is already producing resistant microbes. Their overuse in animal husbandry further intensifies that social crisis. Animals are also used in medical research and as pets. The latter may mean the pet arriving from another country and again increases the risk of spreading disease. For Quammen, contemporary human performance and societal settings are offering irresistible opportunities for enterprising microbes.

The modern world posits historian Matthew Ward (2020) has been shaped by contagions. Plagues, influenzas, and the host of infectious diseases (smallpox, measles, mumps, chickenpox, as well as influenza) that were brought from Europe to the Americas in the 16th and 17th centuries have left a significant mark on today's world. Vulnerable communities and their civilisations were wiped out in the Americas. These 'virgin soil epidemics' wiped out up to 95% of the indigenous population in some regions where contact was made with European traders and invaders. The collective memory of the affected communities also disappeared. These peoples were pre-literate. Knowledge was retained by elders. It was retrieved by the next generation only by listening to the experiences and folklore passed to them through the telling of stories. Ward remarks that those who survived the disease were left in despair.

COVID-19 will have a long-term effect on the future shape of global society, Ward notes, but the future will be shaped is yet unknown. What is known is that humans could reshape their relationship with other life forms (and each other) to provide a more certain future for both. If humanity does not deal effectively and urgently with zoonosis then, to put it bluntly, it will add to the already long list of stupidities manufactured by humans.

Disasters

This chapter makes much of material gleaned from studies of 'disasters'. As mentioned in the introduction to the book, disaster is a term I am using interchangeably with crisis, catastrophe, and calamity. However, the study of disasters is a specific academic and pragmatic discipline. Disaster studies have emerged as a specialist subject, combining empirical research and theoretical reasoning from, for example, sociology, anthropology, political science, and environmentalism, with the experiences and policies arising from dealing with mass emergencies (Andharia, 2020). Michael Lindell is a researcher specialising in 'emergency preparedness and response'. His research has covered a wide range of natural and human-made hazards. For Lindell (2013), disaster studies address the effects on and responses of society and individuals from mass emergencies caused by, for example, earthquakes and hurricanes, nuclear accidents, violent intergroup conflicts, and shortages of vital resources (especially food and water). These events can be classified as 'mass emergencies' when they disrupt everyday routines and threaten the lives and well-being of large numbers of people and destroy large amounts of property and infrastructure.

Life on earth has been repeatedly desecrated by disaster. Over billions of years, a churning mixture of atmospheric and chemical cyclical commotions mitigated against any form of living organism existing let alone persisting. For palaeontologist and evolutionary biologist Henry Gee (2022), not only is life remarkable for its inaugurate ability but incredible for its regenerative facility. The existence and persistence of hominoids and subsequently Homo sapiens in the face of dangers and devastations both not of their own making and for which they have been clearly or circuitously blameable is almost inconceivable.

Disasters involving human life, and other kinds of social animals, have a particular configuration. Humans are susceptible to misfortune not of their own making, as are other forms of life, but they also all too frequently make mayhem. A sizeable meteorite crashing into the earth is not the fault of humanity (although such a catastrophic event has become more predictable and possibly preventable because of human ingenuity). But what is the fault of humanity are nuclear accidents and attacks, the spread of lethal infections amongst indigenous populations, and the destruction of the biosphere due to the contaminants of human industrial and technological ingenuities. The old dangers persist, and humans are persisting in creating new ones (Quarantelli *et al.*, 2007).

Disasters are large-scale incidents that may lead to personal distress (physical and psychological), death, and the destruction of property. A social crisis is a disaster that has severe consequences for the structures and processes that bind a local community, nation or broader geo-political area, or possibly the world. But epidemiologists Emily Goldmann and Sandro Galea (2014) recognise the definition of disaster is not consistent in the academic literature. Moreover, the common usage of the term adds to its indefinite description.

However, Goldman and Galea suggest that common features applicable to disasters are that they threaten the resources and/or existence of large groups of people, and they have secondary long-term negative effects on the well-being of the individuals involved. What they do not recognise is how disasters may progress psychological solidity.

Every day there is a disaster somewhere in the world. Each year the lives of millions of people are impacted by disasters. Moreover, disaster incidents are increasing due to human activity. This increase is associated with the spread of contagions and climatic catastrophes, and although interpersonal and international lethal conflict has reduced since medieval times the threat of nuclear warfare with its catastrophic consequences remains.

For Goldman and Galea, there are three types of disasters for which they provide examples: (1) unavoidable natural disasters, for example, floods; (2) unintentional human-made intentional disasters, for example, the 1986 accidental release of radioactive material from Chernobyl; (3) intentional human-made acts such as mass violence and terrorism. However, human activity is responsible for either causing or exacerbating 'natural' and 'accidental' disasters. Today, many floods are connectable to deliberate human activities, and nuclear installations and their systems of safety have not been set up by nature. Positioning populations in locales that are known to be prone to natural disasters imposes extra risks to people and property that are non-natural. Moreover, when the infrastructure in those areas is not constructed to high enough standards to withstand or minimise blows from nature then humans are complicit in the destruction and deaths that follow. For example, suspicions arose soon after the two major earthquakes that struck Turkey and Syria in 2023 that buildings had been built shoddily in a known earthquake region (Horton and Armstrong, 2023). Some newly erected buildings were reported as having 'crumbled to dust'. This was despite there being regulations in Turkey meant to ensure construction companies ensured that their buildings were able to absorb the impact of earthquakes. The question of why the national and local authorities allowed a large number of people to live in those areas must also be raised. Tens of thousands of people died from these earthquakes, and allegedly the death toll was made far worse because of disastrous human actions (that is, building and living in disaster zones) and inactions (that is, not following regulations). Further earthquakes occurred in both countries in the following weeks, killing more people (Al Jazeera, 2023). Some of these subsequent deaths may have been the result of people of returning to their homes, indicating that the authorities had not cleared the area despite the common understanding that aftershocks affecting the same zone as the main earthquake(s) are not unusual.

Most studies of the psychological sequelae of disaster do not address the core cause or cure – societal insanity and societal sanity. For example, pertinent and compassionate interpersonal interventions to support survivors are made by psychologists James Halpern, Amy Nitza, and Karla Vermeulen (2019) who specialise in the study of disasters. They have experience of working with mental health professionals in the aftermath of hurricanes, tornadoes, and mass shootings in the USA, and the Ebola outbreak in Guinea. But no matter how necessary and empathic, these interventions (for both survivors and responders) pertain to the microcosm of human suffering, not their macrocosmic underpinnings.

Another specialist in the study of disasters, Ilan Kelman expresses the macroscopic underpinnings thus:

Disasters occur due to societal failure.

(Kelman, 2021)

Kelman (2020; 2021) argues that attributing disaster to 'nature' is a misnomer. Lives lost, property destroyed, ecological deviation, and the impairment of biodiversity, through hurricanes, tornados, volcanic eruptions, and climate change, is caused by societal disasters. Specifically, the unequal distribution of power in society affects the distribution of resources thereby forcing the powerless into vulnerable living conditions. The vulnerability of being materially and culturally disadvantaged creates further vulnerabilities including contact with animals that harbour diseases that previously had not infected humans and possibly exposure to the leaks from laboratories located in their midst. Blaming nature (or providence or divine retribution) prevents what Kelman refers to as 'real solutions' to disasters.

David Alexander[1] (1993; 2016) specialises in risk and reduction applied to natural disasters such as earthquakes, volcanic eruptions, flooding, and droughts. For him confronting disasters entails accepting globalisation, advances in technology, and consumer culture. He accepts disasters are part of human existence and therefore plans to limit their effects and deal with their aftermaths that need to be in situ long before they occur. Alexander (2020a; 2020b) criticises Governments and emergency response agencies for failing to plan for disasters, and the COVID-19 pandemic demonstrates this failure clearly. Pandemics are predictable, he argues, but not anticipated. Contemporary lifestyles and social systems generate more opportunities for diseases such as COVID-19 to be activated and spread exponentially. As a corollary to his argument that pandemics are societal sicknesses (with concurrent biological initiations and implications), David Alexander (2021) suggests that much of the necessary planning and responses need to be, and usually are societal and not merely medical.

David Alexander submits that no matter the mayhem, the main civilisations can survive disasters or be taken over by other societies. The main exception, however, is a nuclear war or accident if this was to be on a large enough scale to destroy all human life. A large enough asteroid hitting the earth may also preclude the survival of humanity. But in both cases, there may be some forms of life other than that of humans that could survive.

Disasters, for David Alexander (2016), reveal how society is working or not working. It also shines a light on how the way society operates shapes how humans operate. Alexander offers the example of how the embodiment of capitalism, the maximisation of profit, ensues during and after disasters due to the scarcity of goods. But a cautionary addendum to any analysis is offered by David Alexander. Ubiquitous uncertainty and the exponential pace of change mean that any understanding of how society is operating let alone a prediction of how it will do so in the future or any recommendation of how it should function is prone to miscalculation and misdirection. Catastrophic contagions such as COVID-19 exposed the faults in the functioning of global society and also revealed the resourcefulness of its inhabitants.

COVID-19

Contagion is the communication of disease (plague or pestilence) from one body to another body by contact direct or mediate. There is also an implication of moral corruption in its usage. Contagions have and continue to disrupt if not destroy human life and humanity's civilisations.

Tens of thousands of viruses and 300,000 species of bacteria are already known to be capable of infecting humans. Public health authorities and intelligence agencies consider contagions as a threat to global security and social order. Some past pestilences have led to formidable modifications to human performance and to the societies in which they occurred (Byrne, 2008; Cartwright, 2014; Dobson, 2007; Russell and Parker 2020; Spinney, 2018). Smallpox, plagues, and influenzas may have dramatically altered human behaviour, emotions, and thinking, and the course of human history and contributed to the collapse of civilisations (Ward, 2020; Wazer C, 2016; Williams, 2011).[2]

However, the COVID-19 pandemic was not only a biological malevolence but also a formidable and tangible globalised 'mega' societal insanity. It laid bare a series of societal insanities already in existence, disclosed otherwise submerged societal insanities, and created the conditions for the emergence of additional insanities.

As with previous catastrophic contagions smallpox, plagues, and influenzas, the spread globally of COVID-19 in early 2020 provoked both considerable changes to the operation of society and prompted immense reshaping of people's lives (Klein, 2020; Snowden, 2020). But in an interconnected world, this contagion spread far more easily, and its effects were far more widespread. As sociologist and philosopher Slavoj Žižek (2020) notes, COVID-19 has 'shaken the world'. This pandemic seems also to have shaken minds.

The COVID-19 pandemic has perpetuated much morbidity and mortality. The virus's damage and destruction to the body has led David Alexander, to observe:

> In terms of its scope, Covid-19 is like no other disaster that has occurred in the last 100 years, since, in fact, the influenza pandemic of 1918–1920 killed more people than both world wars combined, and contributed to the end of the First World War.
>
> (Alexander, 2020b)

In early April of 2022, the World Health Organisation reported an estimated death toll caused by the COVID-19 pandemic of approximately 15 million people. This figure is the combined direct and indirect excess mortality rate covering the period 1 January 2020 to 31 December 2021. Excess mortality means the difference in the number of deaths that occurred and those expected without the pandemic having occurred. Direct mortality refers to COVID-19 having been identified medically as the precise cause of death. Indirect mortality refers to inferred lethal effects from depleted health and social services whereby existing illnesses arising during the period of the pandemic could not be provided with adequate or any treatment and support (World Health Organisation, 2022).

The COVID-19 pandemic, however, also had an impact on excess deaths in the other direction. Voluntary and involuntary confinements lowered the number of expected deaths from vehicle accidents and occupational injuries. The risk of death and injury was lower when more people worked and shopped from home, used home-based entertainment, and exercised locally. During government-instigated and legally enforced 'lockdowns' whole populations were confined to their houses. But this had a countervailing consequence of escalating exposure to physical harm from, for example, domestic violence, and domestic accidents. It also escalated exposure to psychological suffering due to unwanted loneliness and involuntary idleness. In turn, these negative effects of being housebound and having less social contact with wider family members, friends, and colleagues were mitigated by using digital forms of communication, which proliferated during this pandemic. Moreover, couples and children living in the same household had the opportunity to share and care for each more because other demands on their time and energy had decreased if not ceased.

'Long-COVID' describes the continuation of physical symptoms associated with the infectious stage (Nabavi, 2020). Apart from somatic sufferings such as pneumonia and septic shock, and the risk of death in the infectious stage, the various variants of the virus are associated with a range of severe neurological morbidities. These include cerebral haemorrhage, Parkinson's Disease, Guillain-Barré syndrome, and dementia (Taquet *et al.*, 2021). Cognitive decline has also been attributed to severe COVID-19 infections and may occur even in milder cases. The decline can be significant, and recovery is either gradual or unachievable. Symptoms of cognitive decline associated with COVID-19 include 'brain fog', lethargy, aphasia; reduction in the ability to recall, reason, and problem-solve; insomnia; and inattention. Anxiety and signs of post-traumatic stress have also been linked to deficiencies in cognition caused by COVID-19 (Hampshire *et al.*, 2022). Moreover, alterations in brain structure, for example, 'shrinking' in the overall size, have been correlated with COVID-19 infection (Douaud *et al.*, 2022).

The COVID-19 pandemic caused industrial, economic, political, transport, communication, entertainment and arts, food, and healthcare systems, to be rearranged, ravaged, or re-invented (Berenson, 2020; Horton, 2020; Nicola *et al.*, 2020; Norberg, 2020). For example, some governments used massive amounts of 'quantitative easing' to support employees, businesses, and health services, and research into the workings of and remedies for the virus (Halligan, 2020). Those countries that adopted quantitative easing to prevent or resolve social problems related to COVID-19 generated an economic problem by increasing national indebtedness and price inflation (Tucker, 2022). The invasion of Ukraine by Russia in 2022 further complicated the economic consequences of the COVID pandemic with military budgets around the world increasing. This includes Germany, which has been for decades resistant to funding the North Atlantic Treaty Organisation (NATO) proportionate to the size of its economy due to its militaristic past, which has boosted spending on defence (Von der Burchard, 2022). Furthermore, both COVID-19 and the invasion of Ukraine by Russia raised the risk of nuclear weapons being used on the battlefield and raised doubts about the viability of the 'mutual destruction' compact intended to prevent any nuclear encounters (Hastings, 2022; Research Center for Nuclear Weapons Abolition & Nautilus Institute, 2021).

While some businesses during the COVID-19 pandemic failed, others flourished. The latter includes the acceptable face of business in the form of corporate and specialist internet retailers, but also unacceptable ones such as trafficking women and girls for sexual exploitation (United Nations, 2020a). The pandemic pushed many into poverty but for the wealthiest people in the world it reaped huge financial benefits (Peterson-Withorn, 2021)

Trust during a disaster is vital (World Health Organisation, 2017c). But trust in politicians, already at a low ebb, was reduced further during this pandemic (Berenson, 2020; Rawnsley, 2020; Seyd, 2020). Medical expertise based on orthodox science also endured distrust with 'vaccine scepticism' and 'vaccine hesitancy' rife in social media and amongst local communities in low- and middle-income regions (Simas and Larson, 2021; Wilson and Wiysonge, 2020).

There is, therefore, an ongoing and vituperative tussle about what is authentic 'truth'. On one side there is an affirming of 'multiple truths' and 'post-truth', along with mindful mendacity and downright lying. On the other side, there is an avowal to struggle against 'truth decay' along with the endorsement of truthfulness as a moral imperative (Mertens, 2016). Truthfulness is also considered to be a prerequisite for political, economic, scientific, and legitimacy (Dobson, 2020; Sanney *et al.*, 2020). Psychotherapist Tonya Lester (2020) argues that truthfulness in romantic relationships can reduce the likelihood of them becoming 'insane' by deepening intimacy and improving self-esteem. The search for consistent certainty is therefore considered a categorical cornerstone of societal sanity and psychological solidity.

Scientific knowledge during the COVID-19 pandemic began being paraded in public as personifying truth as never before due to the efforts taken by scientists and politicians to deliver their messages about the realities of the contagion via mass broadcasting outlets. By December 2020, astonishing advances had been made in public health and medical knowledge about the spread, control, treatment, and prevention of the disease (Anderson *et al.*, 2020). But the status of science also came under public scrutiny. Conspicuous contempt based on unfounded and conspiratorial conjecturing abounded especially in social media. These, in turn, have become susceptible to scrutiny and ridicule (Ball and Maxmen, 2020; Borgonovi and Pokropek, 2021; Izugbara and Obiyan, 2020).

These societal transformations and enigmas, instigated by a biological disaster (but one which has societal geneses – as all do), have generated sizable shifts and contrariness in the expression and connotation of behaviours, thoughts, and emotions of individuals. Behaviour, thinking, and emotion are the integrated elements of 'human performance' – including mental health (Morrall, 2017; 2020).

The pandemic may have further fomented an already buoyant contest over what is and who tells the truth, particularly during the Trump presidency of the USA (2017–2021). But no matter the reality of destruction and death, warfare ignites a firestorm of propaganda whereby the veracity of ruined cities and obliterated human life is susceptible to disbelief and alternative interpretation.

Ian Goldin is a scholar of globalisation and technological and economic development. He has previously occupied senior roles at, for example, the World Bank, and the Organisation for Economic Co-operation and Development, as well as being an advisor to South African President Nelson Mandala. Goldin (2021) argues that pandemics before COVID-19 dramatically altered the political and economic landscapes of affected countries in a similar way to wars. According to Goldin, the 14th-century 'Black Death' bubonic plague created considerable shortages of workers to toil the land. This lack of labour, agues Goldin, hastened the end of feudalism and serfdom in Europe. He also provides the example of the 1802 Haitian outbreak of yellow fever in 1802 that decimated Napoleon Bonaparte's army sent to crush a revolt by slaves. This contagion, suggests Goldin, led to the French Emperor abandoning his apparent intention to conquer the USA.

However, Godin points out that the potential effects on society of contemporary crises, unlike those of the past, can benefit to a greater degree from hindsight and foresight. They can be mediated, and catastrophic consequences can be averted or curbed:

> [W]hereas in the past the causes and implications of pandemics were unknown and societies stumbled into the future, we now have a clearer understanding of the causes of diseases and how to prevent them to shape our futures for the better, as we do for climate change and other great threats that we face.
>
> (Goldin, 2021, pp. 239/240)

For Goldin past contagions and conflicts did not need to commence on a course leading to catastrophe. They could have been prevented completely or their trajectories can be interrupted. This is a lesson to be learned for the avoidance of future crises or if not deterrence then the diminution of their impact.

There is an interplay of actual and potentially catastrophic consequences between the various types of social crises. Catastrophic contagions and conflicts risk igniting additional social crises as well as exposing and exacerbating many of society's underlying problems. Conflicts (especially nuclear war) risk intensifying damage to the earth's ecology and igniting and spreading deadly diseases. Changes in global climatic conditions risk fomenting contagions and inflaming social tensions within and between geopolitical regions.

Goldin points to how COVID-19 impacted numerous long-standing social problems:

> [T]he coronavirus pandemic has revealed and compounded pre-existing inequalities in wealth, race, gender, age, education and geographical location.
>
> (Goldin, 2021, p.11)

For Goldin, it is inequality that is affected particularly by social crises. Along with the COVID-19 pandemic and the climate emergency, he cites continuing crisis of antibiotic resistance as furthering wealth gaps. Antibiotic resistance has led to the spreading of previously treatable deadly diseases particularly amongst the poor. Already there is evidence that antibiotic resistance is responsible for making and prolonging morbidity, and for more deaths globally each year than the annual death rate from AIDS or Malaria. The highest number of deaths from antibiotic resistance deaths are occurring in sub-Saharan Africa and South Asia and the lowest in high-income countries (Antimicrobial Resistance Collaborators, 2022).

But for environmental and political activist George Monbiot (2020), this crisis threatens the survival of the whole of humanity. Monbiot mentions that industrial-style farming is based on crowding animals together to maximise profit. This system leads to greater vulnerability to disease and therefore and therefore antibiotics are given prophylactically. In some countries, antibiotics are also used to promote growth in the animals. Goldin (2021) also refers to profit-driven misuse of antibiotics in animal husbandry but adds that antibiotic resistance is increased further through permissive 'prescribing' (supplied with or without medical oversight) for inappropriate corporeal complaints, and their application on the hulls of ships to reduce the growth of barnacles.

However, signs of a saner society were perceptible, suggests Godin during the COVID-19 pandemic:

> The frictions that divided societies (not least in Britain over Brexit) were briefly overcome as families, neighbours and communities came together to address the common threat posed by the pandemic. Health, community and family became more important.
>
> (Goldin, 2021, p.181)

Goldin adds that the COVID-19 pandemic also exacerbated existing and engendered new societal 'fault lines' that adversely affected people. It aggravated pre-existing physical and psychological infirmities (in part because health services became less accessible), raised levels of psychological suffering due to increased loneliness, anxiety about becoming or remaining unemployed, domestic abuse, and abuse of drugs. There was a heightening in general levels of unhappiness and 'stress' (that is, anxiety). In certain countries (for example, India and Malawi), there was a rise in incidents of self-harm and suicide.

The poor, children, young people, and the elderly, and those living on their own, were particularly vulnerable to the detrimental repercussions of the pandemic (Arnold-Forster, 2021).

Epidemiologist with a focus on health inequalities Michael Marmot has campaigned over decades for a recognition of the relationship between social and health inequities. He points out that physical and mental health deteriorates when there is a wide gap in wealth. Marmot also steered a review by The Health Foundation, an independent charity for health care for people in the UK. The review examined the effects on health from the COVID-19 pandemic in England (Marmot *et al.*, 2020). He concluded that those families worst affected by the pandemic were the poor. Not only were death rates higher amongst materially deprived families but their children were left hungrier and unhappier than they were before the pandemic. Other groups most at risk from death due to the pandemic were key health and care workers and ethnic minority groups. Marmot argued that post-pandemic there should not be a return to the status quo regarding a social structure that props up if not propagates disparities. Psychological suffering amongst young people had increased as had domestic violence with women disproportionately victimised. Marmot's stance on shifting the status quo is supported by a subsequent report by The Health Foundation:

> [T]here is an opportunity [post-pandemic] to create a healthier, more resilient society. Government must address the root causes of poor health and invest in people and their communities – their jobs, housing, education and communities.
>
> (Suleman *et al.*, 2021, p.70)

What Marmot and The Heath Foundation are illustrating is the interconnection of the physical, psychological, and societal. Žižek is more elaborate and forthright regarding the role of society in this interplay. For Žižek (2020), COVID-19 was not only caused by global capitalism but revealed contemporary contradictions in which pre-modern thinking about the source and spread of contagions and subsequent systems of social control coincided with instances of ethical progressiveness. The foremost paradox of the pandemic for Žižek is a raising of consciousness about the existential abyss of human existence and the prospect of a philosophical revolution whereby communality replaces covetousness. Locking-up people in their homes meshed with spontaneous acts of neighbourliness.

Predictions abounded about how people's lives and society would change following the end of the COVID-19 pandemic. Writing in 2021, Goldin opines that the tragedy of the COVID-19 pandemic for many people could be an event that rescues humanity. Not to return to the pre-pandemic world would, for him, be a positive sequelae of this societal insanity. More on Goldin's rescue mission is mentioned in the conclusion of this book.

Many years prior to the outbreak of COVID-19 sociologists Robert Dingwall, Lily Hoffman, and Karen Staniland (2012) appreciated that infectious diseases had once again become a major menace for public health. For Dingwall and his colleagues, the social causes and consequences of such debilitating and deadly diseases demanded additional theorising, that is, the formation of a 'sociology of pandemics' to contribute to established understandings from, for example, the medical and other health professions, microbiology, epidemiology, psychology, and public health policy.

Dingwall and his colleagues present ideas that include how diseases, notions of risk (to both the public and the State), institutions dealing with public health, and social crises are socially constructed, methods of surveillance used to monitor the health of the public, the governance of public health, and the responses of the media and the public. Key to the approach of this group of sociologists is the proposition that pandemics are not merely biological entities, scientific and medical knowledge does not simply stand objectively and dispassionately outside the society in which it is housed, and social crises are fashioned not only based on impartial evidence of momentous menaces.

Dingwall and his colleagues do, however, rely heavily on the sociological analysis of epidemics conducted by Philip Strong (1990) to service their sociological enterprise.[3] Strong's epidemic exemplars are the HIV/AIDS during the 1980s and the 14th-century outbreaks of the plague. What Strong discerns is a parrel between when HIV/AIDS spread rapidly across the Western world and when the bubonic Black Death raged across Europe. Both generated profound public panic and were perceived by the public, professionals, and politicians, as threatening the very survival of their respective social systems, especially the continuation of the established social order.

Societies become caught up in what Strong refers to as an 'extraordinary emotional maelstrom' (1990, p.249) characterised by surges of fear, stigma, moralising, and demands for urgent action. Initially, it seems as though the authorities have lost control not only of the disease but of the systems and institutions that service the population's usual existence. Rival narratives arise formulated from, for example, religion, science and medicine, the military, and political ideology, that compete to define and manage the disease and the performance of the public, as well as the shape of society in the aftermath.

While the theorising of Dingwall and his colleagues is perceptive (health and ill-health are patently positioned in a social context) and prescient (they, as had many others, realised the rapid and widespread of these diseases had become much more possible due to globalisation), they do not offer specific preventative or curative actions to combat the realities of debilitating and deadly diseases or the experienced actualities of social reaction when faced with formidable contagions.

Warnings about future pandemics abound and some of those delivering these warnings go beyond conjecture to convey practical and proximate resolutions. Vaccinologist Sarah Gilbert is one of the inventors of the COVID-19 Oxford-AstraZeneca vaccine. Her warning is stark:

> This [the COVID-19 pandemic] will not be the last time a virus threatens our lives and our livelihoods.... [T]he next one could be worse. It could be more contagious, or more lethal, or both....
>
> (Gilbert, 2021)

Gilbert argues for a level of preparedness to deal with coming contagions that matches spending on defence, diplomacy, and the intelligence services. This preparedness, she argues, needs investment in people, research, and manufacturing, so that vaccines can be available immediately. Gilbert does recognise that there are other social crises apart from contagions (she mentions violence and climatic changes), but her focus is on scientific rather than societal solutions.

Plague

The microorganism causative agent of the 14th-century plagues was the bacterium Yersinia pestis. This bacterium devastated the population of Europe where it was known as the 'Black Death' due to subcutaneous haemorrhages producing dark blotches on the skin of the victim.

> The Black Death (1347–1352 CE) is the most renowned pandemic in human history, believed by many to have killed half of Europe's population.
>
> (Izdebski *et al.*, 2022)

But, as with the COVID-19 pandemic, there were social causes to the Black Death as well as consequences and opportunities for society. In the case of the Black Death, however, the opportunities for social change, even more so than susceptibility to the deadly infection, were inexorable.

This bout of the plague is frequently claimed to have wiped out half of Europe's population and all episodes of this contagion to have killed 200 million people. These claims of the Black Death's exceptional lethality are, however, contested (Lawton, 2022). But research using a method described as 'big data palaeoecology' conducted by the palaeo-historian Adam Izdebski and his colleagues (2022) appears to confirm that the Black Death did obliterate up to half of Europe's population. These researchers qualify this confirmation by pointing out that some regions of Europe were not impacted or only negligibly so in terms of the death rate. The mediating factors that led to these regional differences were, in the view of these researchers, cultural, ecological, economic, societal, and climatic. These factors interfered with the dispersal of the *Yersinia pestis* bacterium.

Plague is a zoonotic disease maintained by sylvatic rodents and their fleas. There are two types of plague, bubonic and pneumonic. It is transmitted to and between animals and humans through flea bites, direct contact with infected tissues, and inhalation of infected respiratory droplets. The fatality rate, if untreated with antibiotics, is 30% to 60% for the bubonic plague nearly 100% for its pneumonic variety (World Health Organisation, 2017).

Transmission of the plague bacterium to humans is affected by commerce and communication routes, and climatic and ecological conditions. *Yersinia pestis* is more transmittable from fleas to rodents in warm humid environments. Its spread both in the past and present is linked to particular modes of cereal transportation and cultivation, and to crowded urban areas with poor sanitation. Populations suffering low immunological defence and nutritional deficiency are especially vulnerable.

In every continent except Australia, 'zoonotic reservoirs' of plague are still to be found in rats, mice, marmots, gerbils, and ground squirrels, among other rodents, and outbreaks of plague persist. For example, the plague is endemic in Madagascar, and an outbreak there in 2017 caused hundreds of deaths (Lawton, 2022). Today billions of animals each year are slaughtered for human consumption (People for the Ethical Treatment of Animals, 2022). COVID-19, whether arising from bats or labs, has highlighted zoonosis as an ongoing threat that has and will again threaten to harm humanity.

Historian Frank Snowden records the importance of the plague as a social crisis that heralded huge social change:

> Bubonic plague is the inescapable reference point in any discussion of infectious diseases and their impact on society.
>
> (Snowden, 2020, p.28)

While all virulent pathogens furnish fear, according to Snowden the plague is associated with collective panic, scapegoating, and exodus. Along with widespread debilitation and death caused by Yersinia pestis, these factors trigger an economic collapse and social disorder. The plague produced both private dread and public terror. The 'Black Death' transformed Europe's demography, economy, and culture. Much of this transformation in its early stages was both extremely disruptive to the everyday lives of its citizens and to the stability of Europe's societal systems. But the plague did inspire the development of public health as a strategy to control outbreaks of disease. Quarantine had been used serendipitously and primitively during the Black Death in Europe. But the first quarantine dates to 1377, when Dubrovnik banned travellers from plague-infested areas entering the city. Derived from the Italian word *quarantena*, meaning 40 days, quarantines are a tried-and-tested means of delaying the arrival of a potentially fatal pathogen (Manaugh and Twilley, 2021).

Novelist and journalist Daniel Defoe wrote in detail about the 'Great Plague of London' of 1665 (2010: Original 1722). His account is not contemporaneous (it was written decades later) and much of the detail contained in the 'Journal of the Plague Year is unverifiable. That said, his 'eye-witness' commentary is insightful because it arises from his own experiences.

Defoe's Journal contains vivid descriptions of the excruciating anguish experienced by London's population. People were tormented by the fear of catching the plague and by not knowing how to avoid contamination, tormented by the ineffective and agonising treatments much of, and tormented by grief when loved ones died. These torments were exacerbated by an abundance of sheer quackery from mountebanks selling 'snake-oil' remedies to the desperate when orthodox medical interventions failed to cure or were too expensive compared to the those offered by the swindlers, by the realisation that religious faith was no protection, for those without the material resources to escape the city, an awareness that they were likely to suffer the same fate as those they had watched die a horrible death. The latter was much more likely when the otherwise healthy had been shut inside the same dwelling by the authorities. The practice of interning all of the household when one or more of its members caught the plague was adopted to stop the spread of the disease. But there were frequent breaches despite the positioning of watchmen to block breakouts, and this inevitably resulted in more breakouts of the disease.

Defoe offers rudimentary public health advice for averting such contagions. This built on a belief that containment was possible by confining those who showed symptoms or had been in contact with those who had been contaminated, and seeking sanctuary in uncontaminated locations, did reduce the chances of catching the contagion. This belief was born out of consternation rather than substantiation, and although Defoe's public health convictions turned out to be correct, they were then no more than conjecture born out of personal observations embroidered with journalistic prose.

Those who could leave the city did so at pace. The Court fled to Oxford, and the wealthy to their houses or to those of their relatives in the countryside. Some people who were not rich or powerful, such as servants and artisans, were saved because their services were still required by their employers and customers where they had relocated.

Defoe describes the scenes in the city as resembling a form of mass madness whereby both those unable to leave and those attempting to leave became embroiled in collective hysteria. The population was racked with extreme physical and psychological suffering:

> People in the rage of the distemper....raving and distracted....throwing themselves out at their windows, shooting themselves....mothers murdering their own children in their lunacy, some dying of mere grief.... some of mere fright and surprise without any infection at all, others frighted into idiotism...some into despair and lunacy, others into melancholy madness.
>
> (Defoe, 2010, p.71)

A contemporaneous and much more factually fastidious diary than Defoe's was kept by the English navy administrator and Member of Parliament, Samuel Pepys. Pepys, who lived in London, had begun to write his diary in 1660 and stopped nine years later (Lotz-Heumann, 2020). His diary encompassed the 1665 outbreak of the Black Death, and the Great Fire of London the following year, and earlier the coronation of Charles II (1661). As did Defoe, Pepys records the 'great fears' amongst the population of London, the ineffective 'quarantining' of the infected in their houses along with the rest of their household no matter if they did or did not have any noticeable symptoms, the lack of what later has become known in the jargon of public health as 'social distancing' (for example, relatives and friends of the deceased would still attend funerals despite the authorities legislating against public gatherings), the mistaken beliefs about causation (the most common was that it was caused by 'bad air' based on the genuine noisome odours in the city), and harsh and hopeless remedies. Pepys also makes mention of the 'melancholy' affecting his mind and the mind of his acquaintances, and how the city seemed to have not only a smell of bad air but a melancholic atmosphere:

> Lord! how empty the streets are and melancholy, so many poor sick people in the streets full of sores; and so many sad stories overheard as I walk, every body talking of this dead, and that man sick, and so many in this place, and so many in that. And they tell me that, in Westminster, there is never a physician and but one apothecary left, all being dead.
> (Pepys, 1893; original 1660–1669)

The bacteria *Yersinia pestis* that causes plague is carried by fleas, and fleas parasitically live on rats and the rats proliferated during medieval times because the living conditions suited their existence. However, there is controversy about the role played by rats in the spread of the second (bubonic Black Death) wave of plague across Europe. Rodents and their fleas have historically been reservoirs and vectors respectfully for *Yersinia pestis* in some parts of the world (notably in Asia). Plague remains a threat to humans today because it persists in rodent reservoirs in Asia, Africa, and the Americas. But the spread into Europe of the second wave of plague (the bubonic 'Black Death') may have been too fast, too extensive, lasted too long, and therefore too devastating, for rodents to be the only or primary mode of transmission (Cohn and Slavin, 2023). There may have been in Europe pre-existing human reservoirs and their ectoparasite vectors (fleas and lice), perhaps alongside rodent-flea transmission, that enabled the Black Death to spread so easily to other humans. What could have prevented the plague from surviving persistently in the animal reservoir is the environmental conditions in Europe that can differ markedly from that found in Asia. Human-to-human transmission of plague is far more efficient than contagions housed in the fleas of rodents can infect humans. Humans travel faster than rats (from village to village, town to town, along trade routes, and then off to war), and in general willingly and frequently come into intimate contact with others of their species than they do with wild animals (Dean *et al.*, 2018).

But no matter what the medieval reservoirs of plague were, the disease was to spread easily, as did other deadly diseases, in the filthy, congested, and chaotic towns, along bustling trade routes, and by a multitude of marauding armies.

Medieval medical knowledge remained tied to ancient Roman and Greek notions of the body needing to balance its four 'humours' (that is, black bile, yellow bile, blood, and phlegm), religious beliefs in 'evil spirits' and God's punishment for wrongdoing, planetary movements, miasma (poisonous air). Based on these ideas, medical practices included bloodletting and trepanning (drilling a hole in your head to release them). The plague's course was painful and scarring. Black buboes (swellings) form in the groin and axillae. If these buboes burst, then there was a better chance of survival. Medical practitioners might attempt to assist with that process, but the chance of living was greater if they burst without intervention. Essentially, however, medical 'knowledge' relied on ignorance.

According to biological anthropologist Sharon DeWitte (2014) some of those who had survived the outbreaks of the plague such as those that occurred throughout Europe during the 14th century seemed to have suffered psychologically. This was especially so when they had observed their loved ones and friends die horrible deaths. Others, however, rather than feeling depressed, despondent, devastated, and tormented by guilt for having survived, may well have been elated at being alive. DeWitte has examined the skeletons of hundreds of medieval plague victims and those from the same eras who had not died of this disease. She concludes that the plague was not indiscriminate in its lethal effect. People who already were immunologically compromised, had other diseases, or were malnourished, were much more susceptible to the plague's deadliness. The consequence of their deaths over a short period of time in evolutionary terms, argues DeWitte, may have had a significant effect on natural selection. The plague killed off many of the biologically infirm across Europe and that left the remaining population biologically more robust, the evidence for which is indicated by an increase in longevity. The devastation of the plague still plagues humanity today. It persists as a lethal disease as does protective genetic inheritance but one with a paradoxical import. Mutations that helped people survive the plague have been identified in further research in which the DNA of skeletons found in a London plague pit has been analysed. What this research suggests is that when a person had certain mutations in her/his DNA this increased the chances of survival by 40%. Some of these mutations persist today but they may cause vulnerability to other diseases (Klunk *et al.*, 2022).

Alongside the biological shift were major shifts in the economy and social structure. The medieval economic system and societal power structure based on serfdom if it didn't collapse completely, crumpled considerably. There were fewer serfs to provide cheap or not free labour for the benefit of the land-owning classes, many of whom had also died. Those left were able to demand more privileges in the form of gaining some or more land and higher wages.

The 1665 'Great Plague of London' 1665 was the worst outbreak of plague in England since those that had occurred in the 14th century. The city's authorities did react decisively, and with hindsight, the actions they took were appropriate and would have been effective had they been followed by the remaining population. For example, they ordered the closure of public places such as theatres, and the fumigation of infected houses. Whilst other measures, such as the widescale slaughtering of cats and dogs (thought to carry the plague) and lighting of fires in the streets (to purify what was believed to be contaminated air) would never have been effective they were implemented. Along with the rich and the aristocracy, most doctors, lawyers, and merchants fled from the city.

Public health measures and not medicines have been the most effective in preventing or containing contagion throughout most of human history. The level of effectiveness from these measures has ranged from negligible to moderate, although vaccines and antibiotics were eventually to give medical intervention the edge. For historian and physician Thomas McKeown (1976a; 1976b) the role of medical science was minimal in reducing mortality rates and in England and Wales along with other industrialised or industrialising countries until the middle of the 20th century. People were avoiding early death and the population overall was living longer because of improved nutrition, sanitation, working conditions and remuneration, and literacy. That is, social factors not medical inventions were paramount in saving lives and increasing lifespans during this period. Since then, medical science has been far more potent in mollifying morbidity and mortality, but political, economic, and non-medical technological interventions remain far more effective overall than antibiotics and surgery. The historical accuracy of McKeown's data is contestable, the fundamental element of his thesis persists. Social and physical conditions in which people live and prevailing influences on public health (Colgrove, 2002). Transforming the degree to which humans rely on the exploitation of animals for food, not invading other countries, and reducing the toxic outpourings of a globalised marketplace and travel, counteract and contain social crises much more effectively than vaccines, military hardware, or replacing combustion engines for ones operated electrically. The further narrowing of the medical gaze due needs to be counteracted by a re-emphasis on the sociological imagination and on a sociologically enriched form of social medicine that accounts for biological, psychological, and societal causes and containments if not cures.

Microbiologists, medical practitioners, public health practitioners, politicians, and psychologists, were at the forefront of providing 'insights' for scientific and policymaking and ways of 'nudging' the population towards safer behaviours in countries such as the UK during the COVID-19 pandemic (Hill-Cawthorne, 2020). Sociologists also have something to say about foiling or handling crises of contagion (as they do about conflict and the climate). But Raewyn Connell comments that just imaginative biological technologies and behavioural are necessary to combat contagion, there needs to be advances made in the sociological imagination as well as the inclusion of sociological insights:

Though the COVID-19 epidemic is a social disaster as much as a medical one, and though some sociological ideas circulate in public discussions, disciplinary sociology has had little influence....But we [sociologists] can contribute to responses that mobilize community resources to deal with a social/biological crisis, and prepare for the others that will certainly come.

(Connell, 2020, p.745)

Towards the end of the second year of the pandemic in the UK the House of Commons Health and Social Care, and Science and Technology Committees Sixth Report (2021) remarked that the pandemic had been the biggest crisis in the country for generations. To support this claim the report mentions, the disruption to people's lives through being separated from friends and families, the closure of businesses, the loss of jobs, and the death toll which by then it was more than 150,000 in the UK and globally nearly 5 million.

The success of the vaccine programme in the UK is highlighted, as is the establishment of extra clinical arenas, and the expansion of ventilator and intensive care capacity. But what is also highlighted is the lack of preparedness for the pandemic, the *de facto* implementation of an inappropriate public health policy ('herd immunity'), and the delaying of what were with hindsight appropriate policies to protect the health of the public.

For the Committees, what should have been implemented early in the pandemic was a full 'lockdown', rigorous isolation for the infected and the vulnerable, the closing of the country's borders, and a far more efficient system for testing the population for the infection and tracing contacts of those who had tested positive. What also is criticised is the failure of both the Government and NHS management to recognise the risks to the social care sector when residents of care homes were discharged rapidly from hospital and by not insisting on testing for COVID-19 the staff working in those homes. This led, the report states, to many thousands of deaths which could have been avoided.

Social crises are not random events. There are societal antecedents and aftereffects for all social crises, and Snowden argues that COVID-19, as with all epidemics and pandemics, did not occur accidentally. What Snowden is indicating is that humans and their social systems have created conditions that allow microbes to take advantage. These conditions include humans fighting each other, their misuse of antibiotics, their exploitation of animals, ecological neglect, unrestrained urbanisation, and possible ineptitude in managing dangerous laboratory experiments.

Globally, the organisation of food production and distribution has increasingly meant humans have much more contact with animals allowing what Snowden refers to as 'spillover' from one species to another to become far more feasible and faster. Disorganised densely crowded living conditions have become commonplace in low-income countries and in those where rapid economic development has taken place. Much of the regular business and leisure activities cut across multiple borders and does, and not infrequently people and animals are transported from one side of the world to the other. The regularity of epidemics and pandemics indicates that social crises have become chronic. Catastrophe is no longer unexpected or unusual but regularised.

> Infectious diseases…are as important to understanding societal development as economic crises, wars, revolutions, and demographic change.
> (Snowden, 2020, p.2)

Snowden makes the point that some people are immunologically shielded while others are immunologically compromised. Equally, some people are psychologically shielded while others are psychologically compromised. Vulnerability to infection and to psychological suffering is far more pervasive where poverty, inequality, wars, and the local environment is prone to disaster, are manifold.

Smallpox

In the 14th century and for centuries afterwards, the plague plagued the world. But in the 18th century, Smallpox rose to the top of the most devastating and dreaded list of diseases. It was the turn of cholera in the 19th century and into the 20th century. The bacterium *Vibrio cholerae* spread in humans across many parts of Asia and Europe. However, Snowden (2020) argues that unlike plague (as well as syphilis, influenza, and polio) cholera has a lethal penchant for those living in overcrowded and unsanitary conditions and who are malnourished. While all diseases are to a greater or lesser extent social either causation and consequences, cholera is 'socially selective' and is so in a very specific way. It afflicts the poor disproportionately and continues to so do in sub-Saharan Africa, Central America, and Asia in the 20th century (European Centre for Disease Prevention and Control, 2022).

Acquired Immune Deficiency Syndrome (AIDS) is also socially selective in the sense that certain social groups of people were in the early years of its spread the most vulnerable to infection from its causative agent, the human immunodeficiency virus (HIV). HIV can severely damage cells in the immune system thereby markedly reducing the body's ability to fight disease. The damaged immune system becomes vulnerable not only to common infections but those that threaten survival. The estimated death toll from AIDS so far is 40 million (World Health Organisation, 2023).

AIDS is a zoonotic disease arising from a mutated microorganism hosted by monkeys and apes living in central Africa. The crossing over into humans of this simian immunodeficiency virus may have occurred as far back as the 1930s. The human versions, HIV-1 (the most virulent form) and HIV-2 reached the level of an epidemic early in the 1980s in South Africa and the USA. In South Africa, urbanisation and poverty were major social features of the disease, with colonisation and both apartheid and post-apartheid government policies making the situation worse. In both countries, male homosexuality, haemophilia, and (intravenous) drug abuse were key modes of transmission for the infection, although in South Africa the disease found its way into the general parts of the population far more than in the USA. Globalised modes of transport and migration, population expansion, urbanisation, stigma, ignorance, and an unwillingness to encourage effective preventive behaviours, allowed AIDS to spread across the world from its African origins (Snowden, 2020).

Antiretroviral treatments for AIDS became available in the late 1980s. These treatments to date are not curative, but they are effective in allowing normal life to be led and increasing life expectancy. However, access to these treatments is limited for a sizeable proportion of those affected due to cost and storage requirements, an imbalance in healthcare provision, and sustained stigma (Snowden, 2020).

Smallpox, on the other hand, was more democratic than most contagions. That is, the victims of smallpox came from all parts of the social strata.

Medical academic Gareth Williams has studied in detail the history and effects of what he refers to as an 'Angel of Death', that is smallpox. Smallpox is a viral disease. Smallpox is purported to be the result of a mutated virus in prehistory that infected gerbils. William's research reveals that major and minor smallpox outbreaks occurred from the European 'Middle Ages' (a historical period from the fall of Rome in 476 CE and the beginning of the European Renaissance in the 14th century) to the start of the 19th century. Like the plague, it caused terrible personal suffering and significant social change:

> Smallpox…brought mutilation and blindness, dread and loathing and drove people to inflict hideous cruelty on others. It's impact on mankind was vast, wrecking societies, and entire civilisations and ultimately shaping history.
>
> (Williams, 2011, p.28)

On occasions smallpox had its position displaced as the arch angel of death. For example, in the year of London's Great Plague, 1665, very few deaths from smallpox were recorded.

South and central American populations and civilisations were destroyed in large part due to smallpox, allowing the spreaders of this and other infectious diseases, invaders from Europe to conquer indigenous populations. It also played a part in undermining indigenous cultures in North America. In Europe, royalty and their dynasties were affected by smallpox. The deaths of monarchs and their heirs repositioned routes to power in England, Spain, France, Sweden, Austria, Russia, and Portugal. As a consequence, it shifted the balance of power across Europe.

Smallpox was eradicated at the end of the 1970s except for samples stored in half-a-dozen research laboratories. William estimates that from 1900 to the date of its eradication 300 million people died from smallpox. He also points out that there is sanctification in the scourge of smallpox. Its annihilation demonstrates that it is possible for humanity to rid itself of terrible contagions.

How to protect against smallpox began to be understood in the 18th century. During the late 1790s medical practitioner Edward Jenner realised that cowpox, a minor viral infection caught from, as the name suggests, cows, appeared to provide lifelong defence against the frequently fatal disease of smallpox (Jenner Institute, 2023). In his medical practice in the English countryside, he became intrigued by folklore concerning milkmaids. This folklore posited that, because of their work, milkmaids were susceptible to cowpox but not smallpox.

After a series of experiments, some of which by today's scientific standards would be considered unethical, whereby Jenner used 'variolation' to test this connection, he concluded that people could indeed gain protection from serious disease by accidentally or deliberately becoming infected by a related but less dangerous disease or low dose of that disease. The practice of variolation involved placing material infected with smallpox (such as scabs or fluid or lesions obtained from a smallpox sufferer) on those intended to be inoculated against that infection. Jenner's experiments involved placing material infected with cowpox. What was remarkable about this insight, a serendipitous discernment that eventually would lead to mass programmes of effective vaccination, was it came about at a time when knowledge of microbiology was negligible.

Jenner published in 1798 his research into smallpox with the careful and expansively descriptive title of *An Inquiry into the Causes and Effects of the Variolae Vaccinae; a Disease Discovered in some of the Western Counties of England, Particularly Gloucestershire, and Known by the Name of The Cow Pox*. He had a further insight that remains germane today. That is, smallpox and similar catastrophic contagions are zoonic and specific sorts of societal configurations supply those diseases with the opportunity to circulate amongst humanity:

> The deviation of Man from which he was originally placed by Nature seems to have proved to him a prolific sources of Diseases. From the lover of splendour, from the indulgences of luxury, and from his fondness of amusement, he has familiarised himself with a great number of animals, which may not originally have been intended for his associates.
>
> (Jenner, 1798, p.3)

Tens of millions of people have been saved from premature death by vaccinations have saved since Jenner experimented with cowpox. Vaccinations to protect against COVID-19 alone are estimated to have prevented up to 20 million deaths globally in the year following December 2020 (Watson *et al.*, 2022).

Influenza

Up to 650,000 people die annually from respiratory diseases enabled by influenza. Indirectly, Influenza triggers further deaths from, for example, cardiovascular disease. The most virulent and highly mutable strain of influenza (Type A) is the one that is associated with pandemics. Type A Influenza has an animal reservoir, namely aquatic birds and swine.

Influenza, as with plague and smallpox, has caused widespread morbidity and mortality over long periods of time. Unlike plague and smallpox but like COVID-19, various strains of influenza have spread worldwide. For epidemiologists Patrick Saunders-Hastings and Daniel Krewski (2016) globalisation has assisted and accelerated the spread, devastation, and mutability of influenza and that, in turn, has abetted and aggravated damage to societal systems. This again makes influenza more akin to COVID-19. Sanders-Hastings and Krewski also argue that globalisation has had the paradoxical effect of facilitating international cooperation and scientific innovation to control influenza pandemics or stop them from spreading worldwide in the first place. It is a premise of this book that COVID-19, along with many other social crises, has repeated this paradox.

Influenza epidemics and pandemics have been occurring for centuries. Epidemics result in local spikes in infection incidence and tend to be driven by seasonal influenza strains, whereas pandemics are epidemics that spread globally. According to Sanders-Hastings and Krewski the first pandemic of influenza occurred in 1580. It emerged in Asia, spread to Asia Minor and North Africa, and then to Europe and into North America. Further pandemics originated in Russia in 1729, China in 1781, in 1830 again starting in China, and in 1889 once more beginning in Russia. The most lethal influenza pandemic in terms of mortality has been the 1918 'Spanish Flu'.

Influenza and many other infectious diseases were restricted in their spread compared with globalised systems of trade, tourism, mass migration, and (until recently) mass marching armies. Travelling by foot, by horse, or boat was slow and therefore so was the range of infectious diseases as well as the ability of viruses and bacteria to survive and adapt to more toxic forms. However, the industrial revolution heralded the invention of technologies and machines, and the building of improved roads, that allowed much faster movement of people – and their diseases. These beneficial and malefic interlinked factors stemming from industrialisation fed into the First World War. That brought further technological progress and deaths on a huge scale not just from bullets and bombs but became (misleadingly) called 'Spanish Flu'. The Spanish Flu influenza pandemic proliferated in the poor sanitation, overcrowding, and difficulty of providing effective and efficient healthcare that characterised prolonged trench warfare in Europe.

For Saunders-Hastings and Krewski (2016) the Spanish Flu pandemic is one of the greatest public health disasters in recorded history. It not only instigated severe illness on a huge scale and killed millions, but it changed the world.

The Spanish Flu pandemic is considered to have had three distinct surges. The first occurred in the spring of 1918, the second in the autumn of that year, and the third in the winter of 1918–1919. It was the second wave of infections that caused the most devastation in terms of mortality. There is much debate about the accurate death rate but a range of 40–100 million with possibly half of the world's population infected at that time (Saunders-Hastings and Krewski, 2016; Spinney, 2018). This influenza pandemic was also devastating for economies and armies. A significant number of soldiers and workers were sick, dying, or dead. This was in part because Spanish Flu disproportionately affected people in the 18–40-year age group. Most of those in that age group who succumbed to this virus had been otherwise healthy.

Saunders-Hastings and Krewski point out that if the Spanish Flu pandemic killed the same proportion of the population in the early 20th century as it had done between 1918 and 1920, this would equate to up to 370 million people. Animal husbandry is intricately implicated in the harmful spillover of microorganisms from animals to humans. In particular, it is the considerable increase in the intensive farming of poultry and swine that has made human populations more susceptible to the risk of contracting viral diseases (although not all strains originate in animals). Influenza has been the most conspicuously lethal of these viral zoonotic transferences (Saunders-Hastings and Krewski, 2016).

The geographical origins of the pandemic are uncertain, but it appears not to have been Spain. Suggestion for the first surge centre on either China or the USA. The most severe surge seems to have emerged in Southern England, specifically in Plymouth and Devonport. These coastal towns were important points in international shipping routes, with ships supplying goods to and accepting from many other parts of the world.

The most effective public health strategies were those learned from the plague. The most successful of which was the banning of public gatherings, including school attendance. As with the plague, the public health approach was key because microbiology remained an embryonic discipline (the influenza virus was not identified until 1931). Readily available drugs to deal with the secondary infections of influenza and antiviral drugs to combat the virus directly were not to be available until decades after the Spanish Flu pandemic. Moreover, although Spanish Flu was grave for people and their societies, it had the converse achievement of underscoring public health worldwide as a legitimate and necessary approach for forestalling disease and dealing with outbreaks and increased medical interest in microbiological understandings of and treatments for disease (Saunders-Hastings and Krewski, 2016).

There were to be, however, other flu pandemics. After the First World War, the collaborative scientific reimbursements of Spanish Flu were impaired by a huge growth in trade and travel, and an enormous increase in and interconnection of the global population. Globalisation was underway apace and infectious diseases took advantage.

Asian flu occurred in 1957 and lasted until the following year. It appears to have begun in mainland China, entered Hong Kong, and continued to Singapore, Taiwan, and Japan, before spreading globally. This stain was mild compared with Spanish Flu, causing 'only' between 1 and 2 million deaths, and not disrupting what was becoming a globalised society. By the time Asian Flu got under way so had global health surveillance and medical knowledge about treating such pandemics. That said, another flu pandemic occurred in 1968, this time originating apparently in Hong Kong, and followed a similar distribution pattern to the Asian Flu pandemic. Hong Kong Flu has an estimated similar death toll and also did not result in burdening extensively societal systems. By this time antibiotics were widely available as was vaccination, although public health measures were compromised because travelling by aeroplane had become popularised and the flu virus took advantage of free travel to find new hosts.

Despite the learning that had taken place about necessary public health measures, developments in medical science and associated scientific subjects, and the instigation of international agencies to foster the cooperation that has occurred extemporaneously during disease outbreaks such as the World Health Organisation (founded in 1948), more infectious disease pandemics ensued. These included further influenza outbreaks, HIV/AIDS, and most ignominiously for politicians and policymakers given the readily available knowledge about the nature of and potential for further pandemics by the 21st century, COVID-19. To be fair, global interconnectedness in the form of trade, tourism, and migration, had increased enormously over the decades preceding COVID-19. The Swine Flu pandemic is likely to have originated in Mexico in 2009. This pandemic, which lasted for over a year, spread to dozens of countries within weeks. While public health surveillance and medical intervention had become far more adept in part because of global interconnectedness, a joined-up world also made lethal microbes far more adept at finding new hosts.

This is yet another irony concerning globalisation and the spread of infectious diseases. Notwithstanding the overall interconnectedness of today's world, regions harbouring reservoirs of microorganisms that are pathogenic in humans are not necessarily accessible for public health and medical personnel to monitor and intervene. There is not always the political will to immediately acknowledge the seriousness of infections as they transpire. Also, there may be local cultural norms and understandable fears that mitigate effective mediation aimed at stopping the spread of infection.

It would seem that 'preparedness' to forestall and fight pandemics is either not resourced properly, not properly fathomed, or not properly supported politically. Saunders-Hastings and Krewski, writing in 2016, warned that more needed to be done to improve local, national, and international surveillance, coordination, and resource planning to mollify future influenza pandemics. They add the warning that there would be future influenza pandemics. Both of their warnings were prescient, but it was another virus to that of influenza that struck first.

Science journalist Laura Spinney (2018) recognises that every pandemic is a biological, psychological, and social phenomenon. Spanish Flu, Spinney argues, transformed societies across the world to a greater extent than the cumulative effect of the various outbreaks of plague. She agrees with Saunders-Hastings and Krewski (2016) that this virus was able to take in humans due to contemporary methods of animal husbandry. Spinney also grasps that warfare and the movement of a substantial part of the population from working in the countryside into overcrowded and unsanitary conditions, create the ideal conditions for debilitating and deadly diseases to take hold in the wider population. Additionally, she states that more people died from diseases than from conflict during the 18th and 19th centuries.

The psychological upshot of contracting Spanish Flu and that that of after it resolved could be dire:

> [F]eelings of anxiety accompanied the acute phase of the [Spanish Flu] disease, and there were instances of people killing themselves while delirious. If they recovered from that phase, however, some patients found themselves plunged into a lingering state of lassitude and despair.
>
> (Spinney, 2018, pp.218–219)

However, Spinney does question whether it can be concluded that these effects were a consequence of the infection, the experiences connected to the world war, or both, as they existed alongside each other. Viruses are known to trigger sadness and may provoke a diagnosis of mental disorder.

Temporary psychotic symptoms (delusions and hallucinations) were also reported in a sizeable subgroup of patients who had past the influenza infectious stage. Globally from 1917 to 1925 approximately a million people suffered from 'encephalitis lethargica' (Hoffman and Vilensky, 2017). It remains debatable whether encephalitis lethargica was the sequelae of Spanish Flu, but it did follow a similar pattern in terms of the timing of commencing, ending, the peak in severity, and the overlapping of some symptoms.

Symptoms of encephalitis lethargica included stupor, coma, insomnia, sleep reversal, headache, vomiting, vertigo, dry mouth, hiccups, dysuria, tremors, double vision and other eye irregularities, fever, and a 'mask-like face. Most of these symptoms lasted between 3 and 21 days. However, some patients remained in 'lethargica' for longer or permanently, and about a third died apparently from the disorder rather than influenza. From 1920 to 1924 other symptoms were recorded. These resembled the psychiatric category of mania. Symptoms of this frenetic form included severe restlessness, and involuntary and jerky muscle and eye movements. These symptoms could also resolve into somnambulance. For an unknown number of those patients who survived encephalitis lethargica psychological suffering continued. As with influenza, some experienced what was to become medically identified as 'post viral fatigue'. The number is unknown because it is likely that many who did suffer from post-viral fatigue after enduring and outlasting either or both Spanish Flu and encephalitis lethargica 'put up with it' rather than seek assistance from medical professionals (Anderson and Silver, 2002).

Ukraine

In the top echelons of that list, along with violating the climate and bodging biodiversity, is the conflict humans have with each other that leads to war. Moreover, wars kill, maim, and spread diseases. Smallpox is a prime example of a virulent infection proliferating across countries and continents carried by the soldiers of advancing and retreating armies (Snowden, 2020). The civilisations of the Aztecs in Mexico and Incas in Peru were disseminated by epidemics of smallpox and measles. These diseases were brought into the Aztec and Incas populations by Spanish invaders during the 15th century. The civil war in Syria commenced 2011. In 2017 and 2018, there were outbreaks of measles in northern Syria. In 2022, following 20 years of conflict, a measles outbreak occurred in Afghanistan. The civil war in Yemen began in 2014, and in 2017 a cholera outbreak occurred causing thousands of deaths (Editorial, the Lancet, 2022).

In February 2022, the armed forces of the Russian Federation, thereby starting a major conflict in Europe indirectly involving dozens of countries. For example, the USA, the UK, many European Union countries, Australia, and Canada have provided the Ukrainian military with armaments worth billions of US$. By the end of October 2022, millions of Ukrainians had been internally displaced or had left the country, and thousands of civilians had been killed (Office of the High Commissioner for Human Rights, 2022).

The background to the war in Ukraine is, as with all conflicts (and indeed every other social issue), complicated. In 1991 the Soviet Union was dissolved, and Ukraine became an independent and democratic country. Partly due to high-level corruption in Ukraine and tension between the country and the newly established Russian Federation (especially over Ukraine's improved relations with the European Union), in the following decades, there was an 'Orange Revolution' and a 'Revolution of Dignity', Russia invaded and annexed the Ukrainian territory of Crimea, and long-standing fighting in the east between Government forces and pro-Russian successionists (Mankoff, 2022).

Wars kill, maim, spread diseases, and undermine existing health problems. The level of casualties from contemporary wars is liable to be exacerbated due to the lethality of modern armaments, but modern medical trauma interventions and methods of rescuing the injured from the battlefield have the reverse effect. However, infections such as COVID-19 can spread easily amongst both combatants because living and fighting near each other becomes necessary. Civilian populations become exposed to infections because physical distancing is made difficult if they must seek safety in underground shelters efforts to provide vaccination are disrupted by the war, and both have happened in Ukraine.

Vaccination efforts were already low in Ukraine before the invasion, with only 35% of Ukraine residents fully vaccinated against Covid-19. This low vaccination rate is just one of the health concerns that countries welcoming fleeing Ukrainians need to consider. Ukrainian refugees are also likely to be more vulnerable to infection given their living conditions during their escape. Wars such as that caused by Russia's invasion of Ukraine create crises in healthcare provision because alongside the displacement of a large proportion of the population including medical staff, health systems are disrupted, and health facilities are destroyed. This then puts an enormous strain on the remaining health facilities and medical staff. By-mid 2022, more than 6.1 million Ukrainians have been displaced externally, and more than 6.2 million internally displaced. An estimated 2.63 million of the displaced Ukrainians are reported to suffer from cardiovascular disease, 615,000 have diabetes, 98,500 have cancer, 86,000 are living with HIV, and 13,500 have tuberculosis (Pandey *et al.*, 2023).

The Taliban took control of Afghanistan once again in 2021 when US troops left the country after 20 years of conflict. Two months prior to that, a report was published describing the psychological effects of exposure to violence in Afghanistan during that period (Kovess-Masfety *et al.*, 2021). The authors of the report comment that half the population of Afghanistan is illiterate, the vast majority of women do have not any independent source of income, most people have been exposed to at least one traumatic event, and much of the country's economic and cultural infrastructure had been destroyed not only from perpetual conflicts but natural disasters including earthquakes and droughts. The report's authors conclude that the psychological suffering of the Afghan population is considerable, as it for people living in all war-torn impoverished countries. In particular, there is, they submit, a high prevalence of post-traumatic stress disorder and major depression.

For Snowden (2020) the reason that major disease outbreaks and wars are always social crises is because they are not only medical emergencies. They cause dramatic political and economic upheavals and generalised anomie. There is a breakdown in political, and economic norms, the formidable disruption of normal routines for the public. But Snowden, taking a lead from sociologist Norbert Elias theory on The Civilisation Process' (Elias, 2000; orig. 1939), contagions and conflicts also endow an impetus in the evolution of social life. Examples of this impetus are scientific discoveries, technological advances, and improvements in public health practices. Mass morbidity and mortality engender crises and suffering but also ingenuity and purposefulness. With these observations of the paradoxical effects of war in mind, the social and psychological effects following Russia's invasion of Ukraine will be discussed in the ensuing chapters.

Holocaust

Despite the justifiable attention given to genocide as an example of the dark side of humanity, if not the darkest exempla of inhumanity, the number of known genocidal events in recorded human history is relatively low. Indeed, the word 'genocide', was conceived as late in human history in 1944 by Polish lawyer Raphäel Lemkin. Lemkin (1944) borrowed from the Greek prefix 'genos' meaning race or tribe. He applied the term to what had and was still happening in Germany and territories the Nazis still occupied. This was the systematic extermination of Jews along with other groups of people whose sexual orientation, nomadic life, mind and brain condition (patients in psychiatric hospitals and those with intellectual impairment became subjects for experimental or execution), the Nazi regime perceived as polluting the Aryan 'race' and/or its asserted cultural and economic security. Lemkin was also instrumental in gaining recognition in 1948 of genocide as a crime in international law.

Defining genocide has proven to be a complicated and negotiated process with the need for compromise. Indicative of that complex negotiation is the United Nations Office On Genocide Prevention and the Responsibility to Protect (2023) definition of genocide. It contains multiple elaborations of what otherwise serves as a concise description. Concisely, the United Nations depicts genocide as acts that are intended to destroy a whole or part of groups of people based on their nationality, ethnicity, religious belief, or race. Already in that definitional preface are contentious categories no more so than that surrounding the notion that race is biologically factual, and whether race corresponds to or is separate from ethnicity and/or religious affiliation.

Then there are the difficult issues of which acts amount to the incitement and implementation of genocide and the measurement of intention, difficulties the United Nations does recognise. That said, to paraphrase a popular phrase, if smells, tastes, and looks like genocide, then it probably is genocide. There is no ambiguity in the Holocaust meeting these definitional elements.

There were more than one thousand concentration camps of various sizes set up by the Nazi regime prior to and in the course of the 2nd World War. These facilities of mass extermination and forced labour were built in Germany and across German-occupied Europe. The main camps included in Germany Buchenwald, Gross-Rosen, Ravensbrück, Stutthof near the Polish-German city of Danzig/Gdansk (which had before the war been designated a 'free city' by the League of Nations), and Natzweiler-Struthof in France. The liberation of the concentration camps began in July 1944 when the Russians reached the Majdanek camp near Lublin.

Nuclear

Nuclear disasters have historically been very uncommon. However, their impact on health can be prolonged and pervasive. The International Nuclear and Radiological Event Scale is in seven stages of seriousness counted in 'levels' (there is a Level 0 when there is a leakage or accident such as a fire without any safety significance). Level 1 is described as an 'anomaly'. And is when, for example, there is public exposure to radiation above the annual limit determined in the country where the accident occurs but is not to such a level that it becomes a Level 2 'incident', that is there are minor problems with safety components, low radioactive activity from leaks, or contaminated devices and materials have been lost or stolen. The highest level, Level 7 is when there is a major incident. To date the only two Level 7 nuclear and radiological event has been the 1986 Chernobyl disaster in April 1986 and the Fukushima Daiichi nuclear disaster in March 2011. In March 1979 there was a Level 5 nuclear disaster at the Three Mile Island Nuclear facility accident in Pennsylvania, USA. Level 5 is the release of radiation that has wider and more significant consequences for people and the environment, with possibly several mortalities (Bulletin of the Atomic Scientists, 2023).

The Bulletin of the Atomic Scientists was founded in 1945 by Albert Einstein and the University of Chicago scientists who had assisted in developing the first atomic weapons in the Manhattan Project, The Doomsday Clock was created two years later. The Doomsday Clock represents the probability of catastrophe from human-made catastrophes such as a nuclear explosion that has such devastating implications that the whole world will be affected. 'Apocalypse' is set at midnight. In January 2023 the time on the clock was set by the Bulletin's Science and Security Board in consultation with its Board of Sponsors (that has a membership that includes ten Nobel laureate scientists) at 90 seconds to midnight. This is the nearest to doomsday the clock has reached (Bulletin of the Atomic Scientists, 2023).

When the Doomsday Clock was repositioned to 90 seconds before midnight the war in Ukraine was a year old and apart from a slow-down in the fighting because of winter, there was no sign of it abating in the short term. Indeed, there had been for much of the year-long war signs that Russia could escalate beyond the use of conventional weapons (Dreuzy and Gilli, 2023). Russia has thousands of nuclear warheads, as do the nations of NATO (the North Atlantic Treaty Organisation) although these are mostly possessed by the USA (Statista Research Department (2023). The threat to use nuclear weapons against Ukraine had major implications for the nearby NATO countries, many of which border either Russia or Ukraine or both. Most Western European countries as part of NATO's and/or the European Union's response to Russia's invasion of Ukraine or independently (the UK especially) had and were continuing to provide Ukraine with supportive pronouncements, humanitarian aid, and weapons, as well as denouncing Russia as the aggressor.

Pierre de Dreuzy is a research analyst and Andrea Gilli is a senior researcher for NATO's Defense College. They comment that the Russian invasion of Ukraine, the subsequent warnings made by the President of the Russian Federation against NATO involvement and the potential for nuclear retaliation against the Ukrainian armed forces, was most momentous attempt at political coercion in Europe using such weapons for 40 years (Dreuzy and Gilli, 2023). That is, since the end of the Cold War and the disintegration of the Soviet Union, although nuclear weaponry has been maintained by the Russian Federation and NATO, neither side threatened the other, at least openly Furthermore, the war in Ukrainian and the danger of nuclear conflict destabilised global trade, triggering huge increases in the cost of gas and oil along with other fuels, raw materials, and basic household goods including food products. Dreuzy and Gilli add that the war brought uncertainty regarding the policy of using nuclear armaments as deterrents, the future of arms control and non-proliferation agreements. This uncertainty involves not only Russia and NATO but other countries holding nuclear weapons such as North Korea, Pakistan, India, China, and Israel, or allegedly procuring the technology to make them such as Iran.

The biggest human-made technological disaster in human history occurred when reactor number four went into meltdown at the Chernobyl Nuclear power plant a few kilometres from the small northern Ukrainian town of Pripyat. Ukraine at that time was still part of the Union of Soviet Socialist Republics (Soviet Russia). When on 26 April 1986, the Number Four nuclear reactor at Chernobyl power plant in Ukraine exploded, the fire that followed caused the reactor's housing to collapse, leading to the release into the environment of approximately 100 different kinds of radioactive materials including plutonium, iodine, strontium, and caesium. Within 36 hours the entire population of Pripyat (nearly 50,000 people) were evacuated. Eventually, about 200,000 people were eventually moved out of contaminated areas (International Atomic Energy Agency, 2023).

Initially, two of the workers at the plant died, and within three months of the explosion 28 firemen and liquidators died from radiation sickness or in one case from a heart attack. The firemen and liquidators, thought to be over half a million in number (the exact number is not certain due to poor record-keeping by the authorities), were, in the main, employees at the Chernobyl power plant, Ukrainian fire-fighters, and soldiers and coal miners from Ukraine and other parts of the Soviet Union. The liquidators continued to be exposed to radioactivity as they built waste repositories and safe water systems, and entombed the Number Four reactor in a metal and concrete 'sarcophagus'.

According to the International Atomic Energy Agency (2023), the radioactive fallout from the Chernobyl catastrophe scattered over much of the northern hemisphere via wind and storm patterns, the amounts dispersed were in many instances insignificant. However, the Agency adds that the health consequences from the radioactive material released from the meltdown at Chernobyl have persisted decades after the explosion and will continue to do so for many years especially in Ukraine but also in nearby Russia, and Belarus. The psychological consequences are likely to last longer than the physiological.

Alongside the risk of nuclear weapons being deployed, Russia's invasion of Ukraine in 2022 also risked a similar catastrophic nuclear accident to that of Chernobyl (Bulletin of the Atomic Scientists, 2023). The Chernobyl and Zaporizhzhia nuclear reactor sites in Ukraine came into the realm of fighting in the first year of the war. Apart from the immediate and enduring detrimental effects on health from the release of radioactive material, any major nuclear accident threatens to abate international policies aimed at combating climate change. By 2023 re-investment in fossil fuels had already taken place gas and oil because of the war, and this could increase significantly due to a lack of public trust in the safety of nuclear power plants. Global production and distribution of essential food ingredients such as wheat to many parts of the world would be seriously affected due to radioactive contamination and damage to Ukraine's infrastructure. Industrial and domestic energy supply and transport systems (together with military and civilian zones) had already become debilitated by the second year of the war, and by 2023 they became key targets for Russian bombing. Furthermore, Russia's invasion of Ukraine has exacerbated the risk use of biological and chemical weapons. It may also embolden political and military leaders of other countries to invade their neighbours. Alternatively, it may give those leaders pause for thought given the cost to Russia in terms of the loss of life, finances, and military and political prestige.

The invasion of Ukraine by Russia has pushed the gaze of world political and business leaders in that direction rather than continuing to focus on social crises that threaten millions of humans and the very survival of humanity. It brought a major conflict to Europe but one that has undermined the international political and economic stability, and international norms regarding respecting the borders of sovereign nations. This war revealed how a relatively localised social crisis can furnish a large-scale if not universal social crisis. It is the butterfly effect in action (the idea that a small change in one apparently disconnected segment of the world can, because everything is connected, induce major changes far away).

In August 1945 atomic bombs were dropped on the Japanese cities of Hiroshima and Nagasaki by the USA. Germany had surrendered in the previous May, but Japan was still fighting the allies. The aim of the USA Government and military to drop atomic bombs on Japan was apparently to demonstrate to the Japanese and Soviets the destructive capacity of these weapons. The destruction was so spectacular it could not be ignored by the rest of the world and served the secondary aim of warning potential enemies that the leaders of the country that had developed and possessed them had the will and capacity to use them. The exact totality of people killed in the bombing of the two cities is unknown.

There is much disagreement about how many people died from the nuclear bombs dropped on Hiroshima and Nagasaki. Much of the divergence in opinion stems from decisions about what time period the calculation should be based. It may be hundreds of thousands were killed depending on whether the number of those who died in the following month, months, or year after the explosions are added to the number who died immediately. The number of those who died immediately is probably around 100,000. The disagreement about the death toll also arises from who is doing the calculating. Soon after and in the subsequent years after the bombing, many different groups and individuals have attempted to assess how many people had died. There are the first-hand observations of survivors including local officials and military personnel, and over the ensuing decades a legion of researchers from various countries including Japan, making judgements founded on secondary data and modelling procedures from other conflict events (including natural disasters) characterised by high death rates. The first official assessment was attempted in August after the explosions by scientists from the Manhattan Project. The Manhattan Project was the USA, British, and Canadian research venture that developed the atomic bombs that landed on Hiroshima and Nagasaki. These scientists were tasked now tasked with evaluating not only the casualties as a consequence of successfully implementing what they had developed but every aspect of the aftermath from the nuclear explosions (for example, the damage done to the infrastructure of the cities and the surrounding areas, the effect of on the population in general, and the level of radioactivity lingering in the atmosphere and on the land). Further official assessment of the number of dead was made by the Joint Commission for the Investigation of the Atomic Bomb in Japan, then the Atomic Bomb Casualty Commission, and then the Radiation Effects Research Foundation (Lindee, 1997). The Red Cross, the Hiroshima police, and the United Nations Non-Governmental Organisations Committee have also contributed to the toll of assessments. Another complication to reaching an exact number from these sources is that even the Japanese did not know exactly how many people lived in Hiroshima and Nagasaki before the bombings, and because many different methodologies were adopted. Some sources such as that emanating from the Manhattan Project scientists, did not declare what method they used (Wellerstein, 2020).

What is known is that nearly all of those killed were civilians. Their goal was to have a spectacle of destruction so great that it would not only force the Japanese to surrender but serve as a warning to the Soviets, and the rest of the whole world. The warning was that this new weapon was massively more lethal than any other humans had devised and that the USA was (at that time) the only country with this weapon, and its leaders had the will and capacity to use it against an adversary and had done so even when the military necessity for has been questionable. Killing large numbers of civilians was either the primary purpose of the atomic bombing of Hiroshima to force Japan's surrender and as a warning to the Soviet Union, and the destruction of military targets and war industry was a secondary and morally 'legitimising' strategy, or an accepted collateral consequence. To use nuclear weapons today in similar circumstances to those that resulted in the explosions of

Hiroshima and Nagasaki would not be legal in international law. Apart from the unresolved moral debate and the counterproductive comeback of the 'mutually destructive' defence policy, it would violate the Geneva Convention because of instituting military action knowingly and disproportionately causing civilian casualties (McKinney *et al.*, 2020).

Climate

Contagions such as Covid-19, plague, smallpox, and influenza, and conflicts such as the two World Wars, have resulted in the demise of millions of people but the conflict humans have with nature may lead to the demise of life on earth, or at least most of it.

Incidents of floods, droughts, heatwaves, wildfires, desertification, and insect infestation have increased over the last few decades. Other so-called 'natural' disasters such as hurricanes have become more intense as well as regular. Perhaps the most severe consequence of climate catastrophe is that of a failing system of food production and distribution. (Monbiot, 2020).

These environmental adversities will increase exponentially as the global temperature rises as will their detrimental denouements for society. The pivotal point for sustainable farming worldwide is at 3c above the level before industrialisation occurred in Western countries. At that point, systems of farming are likely to disintegrate especially in Africa and South Asia. Above that temperature then billions of people will be displaced causing immense population shifts as 'climate refugees' seek not only safety but survival. The rise in global temperature exacerbates the incidence and spread of many existing infectious diseases such as malaria and affords the opportunity for the occurrence of infection in humans of novel viruses and bacteria including those of zoonotic origin (World Health Organisation, 2021). Famine and malnutrition add to the vulnerability to contagion and conflict of displaced populations.

Mass movements of people are then likely to be embroiled in conflict as potential host nations attempt to protect their indigenous inhabitants from further depletions in resources. All life on earth may not endure if global temperature rises to 5c above pre-industrial levels (Lynas, 2021).

In December 2020, António Guterres (2020a) Secretary-General of the United Nations gave a speech at Columbia University in the USA titled 'The State of the Planet'. At that time the world was still engulfed by the COVID-19 pandemic but solutions in the form of vaccines and other public health measures were forthcoming. But Guterres pointed to the ongoing climate emergency for which solutions were installed or stalled. He summarised the depth of this emergency in stark terms:

> To put it simply, the state of the planet is broken….. Humanity is waging war on nature. This is suicidal. Nature always strikes back -- and it is already doing so with growing force and fury.
>
> (Guterres, 2020)

Guterres continued with his unambiguous account of the state of the planet with warnings that global warming had reached new heights and ecological degradation and biodiversity new lows. Average annual temperatures had never been higher at any point in recorded history. This is causing ecosystems to collapse and the disintegration of otherwise integrated systems that maintain life on earth. Wetlands, forests, coral reefs, glaciers and permafrost, and deserts are disappearing. More and more land previously suitable for food production and animal grazing is undergoing desertification. The oceans are overfished, choking with plastic waste, overheating, and absorbing so much carbon dioxide that they are acidifying. The annual death toll from air and water pollution is approximately nine million people annually, far higher than that caused by COVID-19. There are more fires, floods, cyclones, and hurricanes, and these are of such a devastating effect that Guterres describes them as 'apocalyptic'. These elements of the climate emergency are manufactured by the activities of humans.

Moreover, Guterres notes that human activity is increasing the incidence of zoonotic diseases, with three-quarters of new and emerging infectious diseases born from the increased contact and utilisation of animals for food, companions, tourist entertainment, and habitat encroachment.

Apart from carbon dioxide, there is more methane and nitrous oxide being released. When high levels are discharged (and they are through industrialisation and farming in general but particularly of animals) these are potent greenhouse gases. COVID-19 lockdowns reduced pollution, but this reduction in human activities during 2020 that contribute the climate emergency only had a minimal if any influence on global warming. Guterres gives the example of carbon dioxide which continued its upward trend despite the pandemic.

The global temperature continues to rise, Guterres concludes, but global climate policies have not risen to the challenge. For Guterres, the science is crystal clear, to stop the climate emergency and the concomitant risk of conflict through food insecurity and risk from environmental disasters such as drought and flooding, the world needs to decrease fossil fuel production substantially. Although this decrease is yet to happen, Guterres is hopeful that it could:

> …Let's be clear: human activities are at the root of our descent towards chaos. But that means human action can help solve it.
>
> (Guterres, 2020b)

There is an emergency but, argues Guterres, there is also hope. Recovery from the COVID-19 pandemic provides an opportunity to make changes in human activity that could prevent the otherwise disastrous upshot of the climate emergency for life on Earth. For the planet to be saved there must be the equivalent of the remarkable scientific solutions and other public health policies, international cooperation, and benefits of a becalmed environment aimed at creating a sustainable and cleaner economy. Deeming economic growth (and particularly using 'Gross Domestic Product' as the key yardstick for that growth) to measure humanity's progress is detrimental to both people and the planet.

Besides the positive effects of the COVID-19 pandemic on the environment, some cities and countries have become cleaner. This is achieved by, for example, controlling levels of travel using combustion-engine vehicles, encouraging cycling and walking, better-managing waste, and implementing a 'circular economy' (based on recycling, repairing, and reusing existing items), seeding more trees and plants, and introducing more green spaces for leisure pursuits and to further capture carbon dioxide and release oxygen.

Guterres adds that there is a moral dimension in the drive for a resilient future. Most of the Member States of the United Nations recognise legally that a healthy environment is a fundamental human right. But for Guterres, a healthy physical environment is inexorably coupled with a healthy social environment whereby human rights, in general, are respected. This includes the availability of inclusive employment, further empowerment of women, and protective measures for those people who are most vulnerable to the impact of climatic changes.

A new world is taking shape and mindsets are shifting, Guterres acknowledges. Knowledge about both what has caused the climate emergency and how to health the planet is growing. More action is being taken by individuals and activist groups (noticeably young people campaigning online and protesting on the streets) to reduce the release of greenhouse gasses. But, while international political commitment is declared, what is missing is action on those commitments, and the need for in-depth and widespread action at a structural level globally is not only pressing but may come too late. Societal systems need to reform radically and the climate-friendly performance of some individuals and activist groupings turn into climate-friendly performance by whole populations.

The year after Guterres's speech the Intergovernmental Panel on Climate Change (2021) declared the climate emergency to be continuing and issued a 'reality check'. This checking of reality included the unambiguous and forbidding announcement that changes in the atmosphere, ocean, cryosphere, and biosphere that threaten the earth's lifeforms are rife, rapid, and rising. Every region across the world is affected by one or more consequences of the warming of the climate. Some of the changes, such as the surge in sea levels, are irreversible. Critical tolerance thresholds for agriculture and health may be breached. Unequivocable evidence demonstrates that it is human activity that has caused the climate emergency. Humanity is on its 'final warning'.

In a report from the United Nations Environmental Programme (2022) titled 'The Closing Window Climate Crisis Calls for Rapid Transformation of Societies' progress on action to deal with the climate emergency was described as 'inadequate' and 'offtrack'. The option of incremental change is no longer credible, the report stated. The only option was prompt and wide-spread societal transformations involving electricity supply, industry, transport and buildings sectors, and the food and financial systems. This report was published weeks before the 2022 'Conference of the Parties' (COP), an annual meeting of politicians, diplomats, and representatives of national governments from most of countries in the world (United Nations Framework Convention on Climate Change, 2022). This COP meeting was held in Egypt. It was the 27th. Clearly, the United Nations perceives the outcomes of the previous 26 meetings have been inadequate and offtrack.

In 2023, the Intergovernmental Panel on Climate Change issued yet more dire warnings about looming climatic doom. There is in this report, described by United Nations Secretary-General Antonio Guterres as 'a survival guide for humanity', the anticipation that technology can be harnessed to help rescue humans from a disaster of their own making. But the main thrust of the 2023 IPC report is that all countries need to implement 'net zero' plans much more quickly than agreed previously in order to secure a sustainable future for humanity. What the IPCC refers to as 'climate resilient development' aimed at rapidly cutting greenhouse gas emissions demands immediate and ongoing action. Examples of this technology are provided by the IPCC. These include the following: using those technologies that produce 'clean energy' or if not completely clean, then energy that produces much lower levels of pollutants; developing further, and employing on a mass scale if proven to be effective, carbon dioxide removal systems, together with planting more trees and plants to do this naturally; making much more use of clean(er) public transport, as well as encouraging walking, and cycling.

Given the sate-of-play of the climate emergency, activist and journalist Mark Lynas, asks 'could civilisation collapse?'. He cites wildfires already scorching areas of California and Australia hurricanes, and hurricanes destroying coastal cities. Any further elevation of the global temperature will result in the Arctic ice cap melting and away coral reefs in the tropics disappearing. From then, if the increase in the global temperature does not steady or subside, food production will falter if not fail, large parts of the world will be uninhabitable, and Billions of people will become climate refugees. If the tipping point at which climate warming can be reversed is passed, then mass extinctions will follow.

A survey of psychiatrists by the Royal College of Psychiatrists (2020) about how the climate emergency is linkable to psychological suffering in children and young people. The findings are that more than half of child and adolescent psychiatrists in England taking part in the survey report that there is a significant degree of fear amongst their patients concerning the climate emergency. Regular 'bad news' about disasters connected to global warming is furnishing 'eco-anxiety' (or 'eco distress'). Common symptoms of eco-anxiety, according to the College, include low mood, a feeling of helplessness, anger, insomnia, panic, and guilt. The College comments that eco-anxiety is not a diagnosable mental disorder, and that worry about what is happening in the world is normal providing the anxiety does not become overwhelming.

Guterres' speech at the opening of COP27 in November 2022 makes it clear that the climate emergency was in abeyance or ebbing:

> We are in the fight of our lives. And we are losing.....We are on a highway to climate hell with our foot still on the accelerator....Human activity is the cause of the climate problem. So human action must be the solution..... Humanity has a choice: cooperate or perish.
>
> (Guterres, 2022)

In a 'position statement' the Royal College of Psychiatrists (2021) claims that climate change, the consequential degradation to the environment and loss of biodiversity, has major negative repercussions for both physical and psychological well-being. Throughout the world, the College attests, severe storms, floods, air pollution, wildfires and droughts, food insecurity, the destruction of habitats for animals, and species extinctions, are altering drastically the ways in which people lie their lives. The College claims that anxiety, depression, and post-traumatic stress disorder are associated with the climate emergency. The climate emergency is aggravating the suffering of those already diagnosed with mental disorders and creating new sufferings which could be so diagnosed. Moreover, not only does air pollution cause physical ill-health and, in the UK alone between 28,000 and 36,000 deaths annually, childhood exposure to pollutants in the air can be linked to mental illness in adulthood. The College also makes the case that humanity is part of the natural world and humans have a responsibility to look after animals and their habitats.

The implication of this position statement from the Royal College of Psychiatrists is that this is a moral obligation to care for animals and the environment as well as a need for such action for the survival of humanity. Indeed, the College makes its moral position clear by stating that psychiatrists and other mental health professionals should champion a model of mental healthcare that is protective rather than only reactive. An alliance of these professions should demand argues the College that resolutions are found for climate emergency, and this demand is 'non-negotiable'.

The mental health impacts of climate emergency are noted in the report from the 2021 COVID-26 public participation event held in Glasgow, Scotland (Wilson and Rae, 2022). Examples of direct and indirect impacts include: post-traumatic-stress-disorder; anxiety and more specifically 'eco-anxiety'; depression; numerous form of addiction including the abuse of alcohol, marijuana, and narcotics; a rise in psychiatric hospital admissions; an increase in suicidal thoughts and acts, and aggression. Increases in air pollution may also trigger and intensify what the authors refer to as 'mental health difficulties'. Societal consequences are also mentioned, including an increase in the displacement of communities and the creation of a category of refugees who are escaping the effects of disasters caused by the warming of the planet, poverty, and food insecurity.

The authors of the report note that the negative effects on mental health will vary widely. The vulnerability of a community to psychological suffering related to the climate emergency will depend on the severity of the impact generated by, for example, floods, fires, hurricanes, and droughts, as well as the perceived risk from such events. It will also depend on how much damage is done to the infrastructure (for example, to roads, supply of power and food, and communication systems), and to what extent law-and-order remains effective. Other societal factors such as the degree of pre-existing inequality, prejudice, poverty, and lack of education, and caring responsibilities (for example, for children, and infirm relatives) may exacerbate psychological suffering. People are already experiencing the loss of jobs, income, homes, and escalating food and energy (gas, electricity) prices (Wilson and Rae, 2022).

Adverse psychological responses when climate-related trauma is experienced for most people will subside when and if immediate danger passes. But for a minority, there is long-term psychological suffering. Incidents of post-traumatic stress-disorder are, according to the authors of the report of the COVID-26 Public Participation Event, substantial.

The actual worsening of the climate emergency together with widely reported incidents of disasters related to global warming, unrelenting and perhaps ill-informed discussions on social media, and persistent governmental and public health warnings, advice, and 'nudging', contribute to growing amounts of fear. 'Eco-anxiety', the chronic fear of environmental doom, resulting in worrying about personal safety, and the future of offspring and subsequent generations, is noted in national surveys conducted in Australia, North America, England, Finland, and Greenland (Wilson and Rae, 2022).

Summary

Contagions and conflicts cause substantial social crises. Over two years, starting from early in 2020, COVID-19 killed millions and made hundreds of millions acutely and/or chronically ill. Just as the world was starting to recover from the severe disruptions to global economic and political systems caused by the pandemic, these were disrupted again when in 2022 the Russian Federation's long-serving President and former Soviet KGB intelligence officer Vladimir Vladimirovich Putin ordered the invasion of its neighbour, Ukraine. But the contagions of plagues, smallpox, and influenza were the mass slaughtering and societal disrupting forerunners of COVID-19, as have been world wars, and will be from the climate emergency. It's as if humanity cannot or refuses to learn from known precedents.

Death and disruption are not the only effects of conflicts and contagions. Mental health is also affected by contagions and conflicts, but not necessarily in such an obviously destructive way or indeed in any way destructive. In the next two chapters, there is an assessment of the validity of these effects and that of a supposed mental health 'crisis'. As part of that assessment the notion of 'mental-healthism' is presented.

Notes

1 There are two 'Alexanders' mentioned in this chapter. For clarification the full name of each is mentioned.
2 There are two 'Wards mentioned in the book. Therefore I have written each name in full.
3 Although Strong's academic credentials are sociological his seminal publication on epidemics is imaginatively sociological, it is titled 'Epidemic Psychology: A Model'.

References

Al Jazeera (2023) Deadly Earthquakes Hit Turkey and Syria, Sparking Panic. https://www.aljazeera.com/news/2023/2/20/new-6-4-magnitude-earthquake-hits-southern-turkey [accessed 21st February, 2023]

Alexander D (1993) *Natural Disasters*. New York: Springer.

Alexander D (2000) *Confronting Catastrophe: New Perspectives on Natural Disasters*. Harpenden: Terra Publishing.

Alexander D (2016) *Confronting Catastrophe: New Perspectives on Natural Disasters*.

Alexander D (2020a) *Building Emergency Planning Scenarios for Viral Pandemics. UCL-IRDR Covid-19 Observatory*. IRDR Report 2020–01. Institute for Risk and Disaster Reduction, University College London. https://www.ucl.ac.uk/risk-disaster-reduction/sites/risk-disaster-reduction/files/building_emergency_planning_scenarios_for_pandemics.pdf [accessed 25th October, 2021]

Alexander DE (2020b) Failing to plan, planning to fail. *IAI News*. Institute of Arts and Ideas, London. https://iai.tv/articles/failing-to-plan-planning-to-fail-auid-1551 [accessed 25th October, 2021]

Alexander D (2021) David Alexander – Key Aspects of Emergency Planning and Management for Viral Pandemics. https://www.youtube.com/watch?v=qmq4JD61iTE [accessed 19th April, 2022]

Anderson K and Silver J (2002) Violence and the Brain. In: Ramachandran V (editor) *Encyclopedia of the Human Brain: Volume 1*. Cambridge, MA: Academic Press. Chapter 217, pp.701–718.

Anderson R, Vegvari C, Truscott J and Collyer B (2020) *Challenges in Creating Herd Immunity to SARS-CoV-2 Infection by Mass Vaccination. The Lancet*, 396(10263), pp.1614–1616.

Andharia J (2020) (editor) *Disaster Studies. Disaster Studies and Management*. Singapore: Springer.

Antimicrobial Resistance Collaborators (2022) Global Burden of Bacterial Antimicrobial Resistance in 2019: A Systematic Analysis. The Lancet, 19th January. https://www.thelancet.com/journals/lancet/article/PIIS0140-6736(21)02724-0/fulltext [accessed 2nd February, 2022]

Arnold-Forster A (2021) Coronavirus: The Price of Global Pandemic Responses Has Been to Make Many Other Diseases Worse. The Conversation, 24th February. https://

theconversation.com/coronavirus-the-price-of-global-pandemic-responses-has-been-to-make-many-other-diseases-worse-155608 [accessed 25th February, 2021]

Ball P and Maxmen A (2020) The Epic Battle Against Coronavirus Misinformation and Conspiracy Theories. *Nature*, 581, pp.371–374.

Berenson A (2020) *Unreported Truths about COVID-19 and Lockdowns*. New Providence, NJ: Bowker.

Borgonovi F and Pokropek A. (2021) Can We Rely on Trust in Science to Beat the COVID-19 Pandemic? PsyArXIV, 21st May. https://doi.org/10.31234/osf.io/yq287 [accessed 31st July, 2023]

Byrne J (Ed.) (2008) *Encyclopedia of Pestilence, Pandemics, and Plagues*. Westport, CT: Greenwood.

Cartwright F (2014) *Disease and History* (second edition). Stroud: Sutton.

Cohn S and Slavin P (2023) The Black Death May Not Have Been Spread by Rats After All. The Conversation, 18th January. https://theconversation.com/the-black-death-may-not-have-been-spread-by-rats-after-all-196521 [accessed 22nd January, 2023]

Colgrove J (2002) The McKeown Thesis: A Historical Controversy and Its Enduring Influence. *American Journal of Public Health*, 92(5), pp.725–729.

Connell R (2020) COVID-19/Sociology. *Journal of Sociology*, 56(4), pp.745–751.

Dean K, Krauer F, Walløe L and Schmid B (2018) Human Ectoparasites and the Spread of Plague in Europe During the Second Pandemic. *Proceedings of the National Academy of Sciences of the United States of America*, 115(6), pp.1304–1309.

Defoe D (2010) *A Journal of the Plague Year*. Oxford: Oxford University Press. [Original 1722: Defoe D, *Being Observations or Memorials of the Most Remarkable Occurrences, as Well Publick as Private, Which Happened in London During the Last Great Visitation in 1665*, London: Nutt, Roberts, Dodd and Graves].

DeWitte S (2014) The Anthropology of Plague: Insights from Bioarcheological Analyses of Epidemic Cemeteries. *The Medieval Globe*, 1(1), Article 6. https://scholarworks.wmich.edu/cgi/viewcontent.cgi?article=1012&context=tmg [accessed 25th September, 2021]

Dingwall R, Hoffman L and Staniland K (2012) Introduction: Why a Sociology of Pandemics? *Sociology of Health & Illness*, 35(2), pp.167–173.

Dobson M (2007) *Disease: The Story of Disease and Mankind's Continuing Struggle against It*. London: Quercus.

Dobson G (2020) Science and the War on Truth and Coronavirus. *Frontiers in Medicine*, 7(563). https://www.frontiersin.org/articles/10.3389/fmed.2020.00563/full [accessed 31st July, 2023]

Douaud G, Lee S, Alfaro-Almagro F, Arthofer C, Wang C, McCarthy P, Lange F, Andersson J, Griffanti L, Duff E, Jbabdi S, Taschler B, Keating P, Winkler A, Collins R, Matthews P, Alle N, Miller K, Nichols T and Smith S (2022) SARS-CoV-2 is Associated with Changes in Brain Structure in UK Biobank. *Nature*, 604(7907), pp.697–707.

Dreuzy P and Gilli A (2023) Russia's Nuclear Coercion in Ukraine. NATO Review, 29th November. https://www.nato.int/docu/review/articles/2022/11/29/russias-nuclear-coercion-in-ukraine/index.html [accessed 25th January, 2023]

Editorial, the Lancet (2022). War and Infectious Diseases: Brothers in Arms. *The Lancet Infectious Diseases*, 22(5), p.563.

Elias N (2000) (revised edition) *The Civilizing Process. Sociogenetic and Psychogenetic Investigations*. Oxford: Blackwell. Original: Elias N (1939) *Über den Prozeß der Zivilisation. Soziogenetische und psychogenetische Untersuchungen*. Basel, Switzerland: Verlag Haus zum Falken.

European Centre for Disease Prevention and Control (2022) *Cholera Worldwide Overview*. Stockholm: ECDPC, European Union. https://www.ecdc.europa.eu/en/all-topics-z/cholera/surveillance-and-disease-data/cholera-monthly [accessed 4th April, 2022]

Gee H (2022) *A (Very) Short History of Life*. London: Pan Macmillan.

Gilbert S (2021) *Professor Dame Sarah Gilbert Delivers 44th Dimbleby Lecture*. University of Oxford News and Events. https://www.ox.ac.uk/news/2021-12-07-professor-dame-sarah-gilbert-delivers-44th-dimbleby-lecture [accessed 20th October, 2022]

Goldin I (2021) *Rescue: From Global Crisis to a Better World*. London: Spectre.

Goldman E and Galea S (2014) Mental Health Consequences of Disasters. *Annual Review of Public Health*, 35, pp.169–183.

Guterres A (2020a) *The Secretary-General Address at Columbia University: 'The State of the Planet'*. New York: United Nations https://www.un.org/sites/un2.un.org/files/2020/12/sgspeech-the-state-of-planet.pdf [accessed 1st August, 2023]

Guterres A (2020b) State of the Planet [transcript of Secretary-General of the United Nations Address at Columbia University, 2nd December 2020] https://www.un.org/sg/en/content/sg/speeches/2020-12-02/address-columbia-university-the-state-of-the-planet [accessed 23rd September, 2022]

Guterres A (2022) *Secretary-General's Remarks to High-Level Opening of COP27*. New York: United Nations. https://www.un.org/sg/en/content/sg/speeches/2022-11-07/secretary-generals-remarks-high-level-opening-of-cop27 [accessed 8th April, 2023]

Halligan L (2020) COVID Has Left Britain Printing Money Like Never Before. The Spectator, 20th November. https://life.spectator.co.uk/articles/covid-has-sparked-a-quantitative-easing-spree-that-could-cost-investors/ [accessed 10th December, 2020]

Halpern J, Nitza A and Vermeulen K (2019) (editors) *Disaster Mental Health Case Studies*. Chichester: Routledge.

Hampshire A, Chatfield D, Manktelow A, Jolly A, Trender T, Hellyer P, Giovane M, Newcombe V, Outtrim J, Warne B, Bhatti J, Pointon L, Elmer A, Sithole N, Bradley J, Kingston N, Sawcer S, Bullmore E, Rowe J and Menon D (2022) Multivariate Profile and Acute-Phase Correlates of Cognitive Deficits in a COVID-19 Hospitalised Cohort. *eClinicalMedicine*, 47 (101417). https://www.thelancet.com/journals/eclinm/article/PIIS2589-5370(22)00147-X/fulltext [accessed 7th May, 2022]

Hastings M (2022) With Nuclear Threat, Putin Makes the Unthinkable a Possibility. Bloomberg, 27th March. https://www.bloomberg.com/opinion/articles/2022-03-27/max-hastings-putin-s-nuclear-threat-against-ukraine-is-serious [accessed 23rd April, 2022]

Hill-Cawthorne G (2020) *COVID-19: Insights from Behavioural Science*. London: UK Parliament. https://post.parliament.uk/covid-19-insights-from-behavioural-science/ [accessed 3rd November, 2020]

Hoffman L and Vilensky J (2017) Encephalitis Lethargica: 100 Years After the Epidemic. *Brain*, 140(8), pp.2246–2251.

Horton J and Armstrong W (2023) Turkey Earthquake: Why Did So Many Buildings Collapse? *BBC News – Reality Check*, 9th February. https://www.bbc.co.uk/news/64568826 [accessed 17th February, 2023]

Horton R (2020) *The COVID-19 Catastrophe: What's Gone Wrong and How to Stop It Happening Again*. Cambridge: Polity.

House of Commons Health and Social Care, and Science and Technology Committees (2021) *Coronavirus: Lessons Learned to Date – Sixth Report of the Health and Social Care Committee and Third Report of the Science and Technology Committee of Session 2021–22*. London: House of commons.

Intergovernmental Panel on Climate Change (2021) *Climate Change 2021: The Physical Science Basis. Contribution of Working Group I to the Sixth Assessment Report of the Intergovernmental Panel on Climate Change*. Geneva: Intergovernmental Panel on Climate Change.

Intergovernmental Panel on Climate Change (2023) Synthesis of the IPCC Sixth Assessment Report (AR6). United Nations. https://report.ipcc.ch/ar6syr/pdf/IPCC_AR6_SYR_SPM.pdf [accessed 20th March, 2023].

International Atomic Energy Agency (2023) Frequently Asked Chernobyl Questions. https://www.iaea.org/newscenter/focus/chernobyl/faqs [accessed 27th January, 2023]

International Rescue Committee (2022) *2022 Report – Emergency Watchlist: Systems Failure*. New York: International Rescue Committee.

Izdebski A *et al.* [62 authors in total] (2022) Palaeoecological Data Indicates Land-Use Changes Across Europe Linked to Spatial Heterogeneity in Mortality During the Black Death Pandemic. *Nature Ecology & Evolution*, 6(3), pp.297–306.

Izugbara I and Obiyan M (2020) Why More Must Be Done to Fight Bogus COVID-19 Cure Claims. The Conversation, 17th May. https://theconversation.com/why-more-must-be-done-to-fight-bogus-covid-19-cure-claims-138220 [accessed 12th June, 2020]

Jenner E (1798) *An Inquiry into the Causes and Effects of Variolae Vaccinae – A Disease Discovered in Some of the Western Countries of England, Particularly Gloucestershire, and Known by the Name of Cow Pox*. London: Law, Murray and Highley.

Jenner Institute (2023) *About Edward Jenner*. Oxford: Jenner Institute. https://www.jenner.ac.uk/about/edward-jenner [accessed 1st August, 2023]

Kelman L (2020) *Disaster by Choice: How Our Actions Turn Natural Hazards Into Catastrophes*. Oxford: Oxford University Press.

Kelman L (2021) 'Natural' Disasters Are Due To Societal Failures – So, Here's a Six-Point Pandemic Recovery Plan. The Conversation, 21st June. https://theconversation.com/natural-disasters-are-due-to-societal-failures-so-heres-a-six-point-pandemic-recovery-plan-161719 [accessed 18th April, 2022]Klein N (2020) 'We must not return to the pre-Covid status quo, only worse'. Quoted by Viner K [interview]. *The Guardian*, 13th July.

Klunk J et al. (31 authors) (2022) Evolution of Immune Genes is Associated with the Black Death. Nature, 19th October. https://www.nature.com/articles/s41586-022-05349-x [accessed 4th November, 2022]

Kovess-Masfety V, Keyes K, Karam E, Sabawoon A and Sarwari B (2021) A National Survey on Depressive and Anxiety Disorders in Afghanistan: A Highly Traumatized Population. *BioMed Central Psychiatry*, 21(314). https://bmcpsychiatry.biomedcentral.com/articles/10.1186/s12888-021-03273-4 [accessed 20th August, 2021).

Lawton G (2022) Return of the Plague. *New Scientist*, 254(3388), pp.48–51.

Lemkin R (1944) *Axis Rule in Occupied Europe*. Washington, DC: Endowment for International Peace.

Lester S (2020) Committing to Honesty in Your Relationship. Psychology Today, 28th September. https://www.psychologytoday.com/us/blog/staying-sane-inside-insanity/202009/committing-honesty-in-your-relationship [accessed 6th April, 2021]

Lindee S (1997) (second edition) *Suffering Made Real: American Science and the Survivors at Hiroshima*. Chicago: University of Chicago Press.

Lindell MK (2013) Disaster studies. *Current Sociology*, 61(5–6), pp.797–825.

Lotz-Heumann U (2020) Diary of Samuel Pepys Shows How Life Under the Bubonic Plague Mirrored Today's Pandemic. The Conversation, 24th April. https://theconversation.com/diary-of-samuel-pepys-shows-how-life-under-the-bubonic-plague-mirrored-todays-pandemic-136222 [accessed 13th October, 2020]

Lovejoy T (2021) Nature, COVID-19, Disease Prevention, and Climate Change. *Biological Conservation*, 261(109213). https://www.ncbi.nlm.nih.gov/pmc/articles/PMC8445747/ [accessed 27th April, 2023]

Lynas M (2021) *Our Final Warning: Six Degrees of Climate Emergency*. London: Fourth Estate.

Manaugh G and Twilley N (2021) *Until Proven Safe: The History and Future of Quarantine*. New York: Pan Macmillan.

Mankoff J (2022) Russia's War in Ukraine Identity, History, and Conflict. Center for Stategic & International Studies. https://www.csis.org/analysis/russias-war-ukraine-identity-history-and-conflict [accessed 4th November, 2022]

Marmot M, Allen J, Goldblatt P, Herd E, Morrison J (2020) *Build Back Fairer: The COVID-19 Marmot Review: The Pandemic, Socioeconomic and Health Inequalities in England*. London: Institute of Health Equity.

Maron D (2020) 'Wet Markets' Likely Launched the Coronavirus. Here's What You Need to Know. National Geographic, 15th April. https://www.nationalgeographic.com/animals/article/coronavirus-linked-to-chinese-wet-markets [accessed 17th July, 2022]McKeown T (1976a) *The Modern Rise of Population*. New York: Academic Press.

McKeown T (1976b) *The Role of Medicine: Dream, Mirage, or Nemesis?* London: Nuffield Provincial Hospitals Trust.

McKinney K, Sagan S and Weiner A (2020) Why the Atomic Bombing of Hiroshima Would Be Illegal Today. *Bulletin of the Atomic Scientists*, 76(4), pp.157–165.

Mertens T (2016) On Kant's Duty to Speak the Truth. *Kantian Review*, 21(1), pp.27–51.

Monbiot G (2020) Covid-19 is Nature's Wake-up Call to Complacent Civilisation. The Guardian, 25th March. https://www.theguardian.com/commentisfree/2020/mar/25/covid-19-is-natures-wake-up-call-to-complacent-civilisation. [accessed 16th April, 2020]

Morrall P (2017) *Madness: Ideas about Insanity*. Abingdon: Routledge.

Morrall P (2020) *Insane Society: A Sociology of Mental Health*. Abingdon: Routledge.

Nabavi N (2020) Long Covid: How to Define It and How to Manage It. *British Medical Journal*, 370, p. m3489, 7th September. https://www.bmj.com/content/370/bmj.m3489

Nicola M, Alsafi Z, Sohrabi C, Kerwan A, Al-Jabir,d A, Iosifidis C, Agha M and Aghaf R (2020) The Socio-Economic Implications of the Coronavirus Pandemic (COVID-19): A Review. *International Journal of Surgery*, 78, pp.185–193.

Norberg J (2020) The Covid Trap: Will Society Ever Open Up Again? *The Spectator*, 5th September. https://www.spectator.co.uk/article/the-covid-trap-will-society-ever-open-up-again [accessed 10th September, 2020].

Office of the High Commissioner for Human Rights (2022) Ukraine: Civilian Casualty Update 31 October. https://www.ohchr.org/en/news/2022/10/ukraine-civilian-casualty-update-31-october-2022 [accessed 4th November, 2022]

Pandey A, Wells C, Stadnytskyi V, Moghadas M, Marathe M, Sah P, Crystal W, Meyers L, Singer B, Nesterova O and Galvani A (2023) Disease Burden Among Ukrainians Forcibly Displaced by the 2022 Russian Invasion. *Population Biology*

Demography, 120(8). https://www.pnas.org/doi/pdf/10.1073/pnas.2215424120 [accessed 16th April, 2023]

People for the Ethical Treatment of Animals (2022) Animals Used for Food. https://www.peta.org/issues/animals-used-for-food/ [accessed 4th April, 2022]

Pepys S (1893; original 1660–1669) In: The Diary of Samuel Pepys. https://www.gutenberg.org/files/4200/4200-h/4200-h.htm [accessed 23rd October, 2022]

Peterson-Withorn C (2021) How Much Money America's Billionaires Have Made During The Covid-19 Pandemic. Forbes Magazine, 30th April. https://www.forbes.com/sites/chasewithorn/2021/04/30/american-billionaires-have-gotten-12-trillion-richer-during-the-pandemic/?sh=79935983f557 [accessed 6th April, 2022]

Quammen D (2012) *Spillover: Animal Infections and the Next Human Pandemic.* London: Vintage.

Quarantelli E, Lagadec P and Boin A (2007) A Heuristic Approach to Future Disasters and Crises: New, Old, and In-Between Types. In: Havidan R, Enrico Q, Russell D (editors) *Handbook of Disaster Research*. New York: Springer. Chapter 2, pp.16–41.

Rawnsley A (2020) The Weak Defence of Dominic Cummings Further Erodes Trust in the Government. *The Guardian*, 24th May.

Research Center for Nuclear Weapons Abolition & Nautilus Institute (2021) Pandemic Futures and Nuclear Weapon Risks. *Journal for Peace and Nuclear Disarmament*, 4(supplement 1), pp.6–39.

Royal College of Psychiatrists (2020) The Climate Crisis Is Taking a Toll on The Mental Health of Children and Young People. Royal College of Psychiatrists Online News, 20th November. https://www.rcpsych.ac.uk/news-and-features/latest-news/detail/2020/11/20/the-climate-crisis-is-taking-a-toll-on-the-mental-health-of-children-and-young-people [accessed 23rd December, 2020]

Royal College of Psychiatrists (2021) *Our Planet's Climate and Ecological Emergency.* Position Statement PS03/2, May 2021. London: Royal College of Psychiatrists.

Russell E and Parker M (2020) How Pandemics Past and Present Fuel the Rise of Large Companies. The Conversation, 3rd June. https://theconversation.com/how-pandemics-past-and-present-fuel-the-rise-of-large-companies-137732 [accessed 13th August, 2020]

Sanney K, Trautman L, Yordy E, Cowart Y and Sewell D (2020). The Importance of Truth Telling and Trust. *Journal of Legal Studies Education*, 37(1), pp.7–36.

Saunders-Hastings P and Krewski D (2016) Reviewing the History of Pandemic Influenza: Understanding Patterns of Emergence and Transmission. *Pathogens* 5(4), p.66. https://doi.org/10.3390/pathogens5040066 [accessed 27th October, 2022]

Seyd B (2020) Coronavirus: Trust in Political Figures is at a Low Just as they Need Citizens to Act on Their Advice. The Conversation, 11th March. https://theconversation.com/coronavirus-trust-in-political-figures-is-at-a-low-just-as-they-need-citizens-to-act-on-their-advice-133284 [accessed 14th June, 2020].

Simas C and Larson H (2021) Overcoming Vaccine Hesitancy in Low-Income and Middle-Income Regions. *Nature Reviews Disease Primers*, 7(41). https://www.nature.com/articles/s41572-021-00279-w [accessed 23rd April, 2022]

Snowden F (2020) *Epidemics and Society: From the Black Death to the Present.* New Haven, CT: Yale University.

Spinney L (2018) *Pale Rider: The Spanish Flu of 1918 and How It Changed the World.* London: Vintage.

Statista Research Department (2023) Number of Nuclear Warheads Stockpiled by NATO and Russia as of 2022, by Type. Statista, 3rd June. https://www.statista.

com/statistics/1309468/nuclear-warhead-comparison-nato-russia-type/ [accessed 25th January, 2023]

Strong P (1990) Epidemic Psychology: A Model. *Sociology of Health and Illness*, 12(3), pp.249–259.

Suleman M, Sonthalia S, Webb C, Tinson A, Kane M, Bunbury S, Finch D and Bibby J (2021) *Unequal Pandemic, Fairer Recovery: The COVID-19 Impact Inquiry Report*. London: The Health Foundation.

Taquet M, Geddes J, Husain M, Luciano S and Harrison P (2021) 6-Month Neurological and Psychiatric Outcomes in 236379 Survivors of COVID-19: a Retrospective Cohort Study Using Electronic Health Records. 6th April, Lancet Psychiatry. https://www.thelancet.com/journals/lanpsy/article/PIIS2215-0366(21)00084-5/fulltext [accessed 7th April, 2021]

Tucker P (2022) *Quantitative Easing, Monetary Policy Implementation and the Public Finances*. London: Institute for Fiscal Studies.

United Nations (2020a) COVID-19 Worsening Gender-Based Violence, Trafficking Risk, for Women and Girls. New York: United Nations News, Global Perspective Human Stories, 30th November. https://news.un.org/en/story/2020/11/1078812 [accessed 10th December, 2020]

United Nations Climate Change (2022) Sharm El-Sheikh Climate Change Conference – November 2022 [COP27]. United Nations Framework Convention on Climate Change. https://unfccc.int/cop27 [accessed 7th November, 2022]

United Nations Department of Economic and Social Affairs (2022) World Economic Situation and Prospects: April 2022 Briefing, No. 159. New York: United Nations. https://www.un.org/development/desa/dpad/publication/world-economic-situation-and-prospects-april-2022-briefing-no-159 / [accessed 27th August, 2022]

United Nations Environmental Programme (2022) *The Closing Window Climate Crisis Calls for Rapid Transformation of Societies*. Nairobi: United Nations Environmental Programme.

United Nations Office on Genocide Prevention and the Responsibility to Protect (2023) Genocide: Background and Definition. New York: United Nations. https://www.un.org/en/genocideprevention/genocide.shtml [accessed 2nd February, 2023]

United Nations Water Conference (2023) Stressing Risk of More Suffering, Death, Speakers Say Financing, Infrastructure, Policy Changes Crucial to End Global Water Crisis, as Conference Concludes. United Nations Press Release, 24th March. https://press.un.org/en/2023/envdev2057.doc.htm [accessed 12th April, 2023]

Van de Straat B, Sebayang B, Grigg M, Staunton K, Garjito T, Vythilingam I, Russell T and Burkot T (2022) Zoonotic Malaria Transmission and Land Use Change in Southeast Asia: What is Known About the Vectors. *Malaria Journal*, 21(109). https://malariajournal.biomedcentral.com/articles/10.1186/s12936-022-04129-2 [accessed 11th July, 2022]

Von der Burchard H (2022) In Historic Shift, Germany Ramps Up Defense Spending Due to Russia's Ukraine War. Politico, 27th February. https://www.politico.eu/article/germany-to-ramp-up-defense-spending-in-response-to-russias-war-on-ukraine/ [accessed 23rd April, 2022]

Ward M (2020) How the Modern World Was Shaped by Epidemics 500 Years Ago. The Conversation, 18th September. https://theconversation.com/how-the-modern-world-was-shaped-by-epidemics-500-years-ago-145905 [accessed 29th September, 2020]

Watson O, Barnsley G, Toor J, Hogan A, Winskill P and Ghani A (2022) Global Impact of the First Year of COVID-19 Vaccination: A Mathematical Modelling Study. *The Lancet*, 22(9), pp.1293–1302.

Wazer C (2016) The Plagues That Might Have Brought Down the Roman Empire. *The Atlantic*, 16th March. https://www.theatlantic.com/science/archive/2016/03/plagues-roman-empire/473862/ [accessed 8th October, 2020]

Wellerstein A (2020) Counting the Dead at Hiroshima and Nagasaki. *Bulletin of the Atomic Scientists*, 4th August. https://thebulletin.org/2020/08/counting-the-dead-at-hiroshima-and-nagasaki/ [accessed 10th February, 2023]

Williams G (2011) *Angel of Death. The Story of Smallpox*. Basingstoke: Palgrave Macmillan.

Wilson N and Rae K (2022) Climate Change and Mental Health: Report from a COP-26 Public Participation Event. https://www.mentalhealth.org.uk/sites/default/files/2022-07/MHF-Scotland-Climate-Change-COP26-report_0.pdf [accessed 8th November, 2022]

Wilson S and Wiysonge S (2020) Misinformation on Social Media Fuels Vaccine Hesitancy: A Global Study Shows the Link. The Conversation, 3rd December. https://theconversation.com/misinformation-on-social-media-fuels-vaccine-hesitancy-a-global-study-shows-the-link-150652 [accessed 23rd April, 2022]

World Health Organisation (2017a) Plague: Key Facts. https://www.who.int/news-room/fact-sheets/detail/plague [accessed 26th April, 2022]

World Health Organisation (2017b) Up to 650 000 People Die of Respiratory Diseases Linked to Seasonal Flu Each Year. Geneva: World Health Organisation.https://www.who.int/news/item/13-12-2017-up-to-650-000-people-die-of-respiratory-diseases-linked-to-seasonal-flu-each-year [accessed 27th October, 2022]

World Health Organisation (2017c) *Communicating Risk in Public Health Emergencies*. Geneva: World Health Organisation.

World Health Organisation (2021) Climate Change and Health; Key Facts. https://www.who.int/news-room/fact-sheets/detail/climate-change-and-health [accessed 5th May, 2022]

World Health Organisation (2022) 14.9 Million Excess Deaths Associated with the COVID-19 Pandemic in 2020 and 2021. Geneva: WHO. https://www.who.int/news/item/05-05-2022-14.9-million-excess-deaths-were-associated-with-the-covid-19-pandemic-in-2020-and-2021 [accessed 5th May, 2022]

World Health Organisation (2023) Key Facts: HIV and AIDS. https://www.who.int/news-room/fact-sheets/detail/hiv-aids [accessed 10th May, 2023]

Žižek S (2020) *Pandemic! COVID-19 Shakes the World*. Cambridge: Polity.

2 Mental Health Crisis

In the previous chapter, the social crises of contagions (COVID-19, plague, smallpox, and influenza) and conflicts (the invasion of Ukraine by Russia, aspects of world war, and humanity's clash with the climate) were discussed. In this chapter, the consequences for mental health of these catastrophic events are explored. These consequences are more far-reaching than how they affect personal well-being. They have implications for human civilisation and humanity's survival. The specific issue addressed in the chapter is, whether mental health can be considered to be in a perpetual state of crisis or do social crises such as lethal and widespread disease, warfare, and incidents of ecological devastation, source supreme spikes in psychological suffering.

In normal times the societal insanities of violence, inequality, selfishness, insecurity, and stupidity, provoke psychological suffering (Morrall, 2017). This suffering is experienced 'sincerely' in the sense that it results in such serious disruption to the emotional stability and lifestyle of the person concerned and/ or to that of others that lay or professional intervention is requested by that individual or imposed by the social control agencies of the State (the police, psychiatry, and the judiciary) possibly at the behest of loved ones. But there are multifarious biological, psychological, and social processes implicated when trying to understand and handle psychological well-being and psychological suffering. Some of these processes seem to suggest straightforward cause-and-effect connections (for example, that experiencing a traumatic event can traumatise the psyche), although even then these would-be 'known knowns' may be affected by unrecognised predispositions that regulate an individual's suffering.

In other instances, there is recognition that there are intricacies, but also an acceptance that their interconnections and trajectories in relation to the cause-and-effect on mental health are not fully understood. These are the 'known unknowns', examples of which include having evidence linking childhood trauma, evolutionary drivers, or genetic mutation, to psychological suffering but this is not incontrovertible confirmation of a direct cause-and-effect connection. There are also 'unknown unknowns', unborn theoretical and evidential understandings, and shifts in cultural values, that revolutionise how particular elements of human performance are categorised as normal or abnormal. It is complicated.

DOI: 10.4324/9781003223757-3

No less complicated is trying to understand the process involved in social crises where the psyche is concerned. Evidentially, some social crises in some circumstances can inflict harm on bodies and minds. Paradoxically, some social crises in some circumstances can furnish psychological solidity (and possibly promote psychological progress). Such solidness may either be innovative or a reification of a latent attribute.

The overarching themes of contagion and conflict are followed in this chapter on mental health. The chapter sections cover specific spheres of conflicts and contagions that have the most relevance to mental health and have been studied the most. First, however, is a discussion of the psychological suffering associated with disasters, in general.

Disasters and Mental Health

The World Health Organisation (2017) submits that certain psychological and social factors will exacerbate the negative consequences of disasters on people and their communities. Pre-existing social problems such as belonging to a marginalised group and living in a country where there is political oppression, a culture of violence, family dislocation and dissolution in a high proportion of the population, are likely to increase the psychological suffering of people caught in calamities. People already diagnosed with depression, anxiety, and drug and alcohol abuse before a disaster are prone to further mental deterioration.

If a disaster is prolonged to the point where it becomes normalised or if one disaster is followed by another similar or different disaster, then what was abnormal becomes a normal experience. Years of warfare, a lifetime of living in poverty, facing daily (and nightly) the threat of malaria, or when early humans had to continuously dodge giant reptilian carnivores, at one time or another have been just the way life was and still is for millions of people. Adjustment to social crises and carrying on resiliently[1] becomes a habit for most people unless the vicissitude is extreme such as in the cases of genocide, nuclear blasts, or inescapable debilitating and deadly diseases and all-encompassing ecocide. This is not to argue that resilience should be admired or encouraged but to point out that humanity as a species has survived this long because it can endure social crises.

According to Epidemiologists Emily Goldmann and Sandro Galea (2014), there is evidence to suggest that human-made disasters, including mass violence as exemplified in the two world wars, result in more severe psychological suffering than natural disasters. Post-traumatic stress disorder was added to the third edition of the *Diagnostic and Statistical Manual of Mental Disorders (DSM-III)* in 1980. The psychological suffering of combatants has been recorded for millennia and in the First World War attributed to 'shell shock'. However, the entry into the DSM of this major mental illness stemmed largely from observations of the psychological suffering of veterans of the Vietnam War which ended in 1975 after 20 years of fighting and the loss of approximately three million lives.

In terms of medical diagnosis, both post-traumatic stress disorder (PTSD) and major depressive disorder are associated with experiencing disaster and may occur as comorbidities (Makwana, 2019). PTSD, as the name indicates, is the psychological sequelae of exposure to trauma. The traumatic events that can lead to PTSD vary considerably as does the degree of stress experienced. There is a higher risk of psychopathology in circumstances of constant and intense exposure to dreadful disasters (Goldmann and Galea, 2014).

The key characteristics, however, are repeatedly re-experiencing the traumatic event in the form of nightmares and/or flashbacks, hyper-vigilance and hyper-arousal whenever actual or apparent connections are made with the original event and therefore avoidance of situations that may remind the sufferer of the trauma including the actual setting. In contrast to everyday misery or 'minor' depressiveness, the diagnostic category of major depressive disorder encompasses deep-seated sadness, loss of interest in otherwise pleasurable as well as routine activities, considerable alterations in patterns of sleep, eating habits, and weight, and expressions of hopelessness that may signify a desire to die. Other diagnoses of mental disorder after a disaster but less frequently than PTSD and major depressive disorder, include substance abuse disorder (mainly in those already abusing alcohol and drugs), generalised anxiety disorder, panic and phobia disorders, and prolonged grief disorder. Other than drug and alcohol, other factors that risk a diagnosis of a mental disorder include pre-existing psychological difficulties (especially if diagnosed medically), gender (more women than men), age (children), ethnicity (minorities), low socio-economic status, and if there is already minimal if any social support (Goldmann and Galea, 2014). Goldmann and Galea list factors as key predictors of psychological suffering following a disaster that may lead to a diagnosis of a mental disorder. The two principal factors are: (1) again the absence of social support; (2) and what they refer to as 'life stressors'. The latter includes the loss of employment, discordant relationships, damage or destruction of property, physical ill-health related to the disaster, and displacement. According to Goldmann and Galea, the longer the lack of social support and the life stressors last the more lasting the psychopathology.

What is needed to reduce psychological suffering and the potential for a diagnosis of mental disorder as well as avoid physical injuries and death, argue Goldmann and Galea, are strategies targeted at prevention and recuperation implemented by local authorities and communities. These should, they suggest, encompass 'disaster-ready infrastructure' such as the building of levees and floodwalls, robust domestic, industrial, and transport energy supply systems, well-rehearsed mandatory methods of evacuating endangered populations, and emergency shelters suitably equipped with water and food as well as skilled staff to deal with both the physical and psychological needs of the evacuees.

What Goldman and Galea point out regarding 'skilled staff' dealing with emotional distress is that the necessary skills are about what not to do as much as what to do to reduce the possibility of serious psychological suffering. They rightly warn that debriefing soon after or possibly any time after experiencing trauma may do more harm than good. Reliving traumatic events can embed associated anguish, worsen symptoms, and inhibit the natural process of recovery. For Goldman and Galea what has become more effective, or at least less likely to be counterproductive, is 'psychological first aid'.

Psychological first aid is primarily, as the name suggests, a short-term measure that can relieve immediate distress by first ensuring physical safety and basic bodily needs are satisfied, providing support by essentially by listening and offering only essential advice such as where to get further help. Psychological first aid is not effective (nor is that its aim) in averting serious psychological suffering following trauma. It does not, for example, reduce the likelihood of a diagnosis of PTSD (Figueroa *et al.*, 2022).

But most people who experience disaster, whether human-made or 'natural', do not receive a diagnosis of mental disorder, and although most people are self-evidently susceptible to psychological suffering if they have undergone or observed killings, deadly disease, a nuclear accident, or an earthquake, most of them will cope. As Goldmann and Galea point out, self-efficacy, optimism hardiness, and adaptability are protective qualities, providing greater resilience even in the face of trauma. I argue throughout this book that humanity has survived so far because it encompasses these qualities along with other attributes that enable not only survival but civilisation. However, both human civilisation and survival are now threatened by the unprecedented impending disasters of uncontainable contagions and climate-related conflicts.

What is missing, however, from Goldman and Galea's preventative and recuperative measures is any sense of the societal insanities that are the sources of most human-made disasters and some 'natural' disasters (for example, flooding caused by deforestation) and accordingly what is missing is any sense of a saner society in which the occurrence of traumatic events and their concomitant psychological suffering is lessened.

Medical practitioner and public health researcher Nikunj Makwana (2019) provides an example of what he considers is the biggest industrial disaster in human history, the 1984 Bhopal disaster. A pesticide factory with the majority share owner the USA company Union Carbide Corporation released toxic methyl isocyanate gas over nearby residential areas. Thousands of people died because of chemical poisoning and hundreds of thousands of people suffered physical injuries. Epidemiological and longitudinal studies of the psychological suffering amongst those affected directly and indirectly by the disaster indicate a wide variety of diagnosable mental disorders and neurological symptoms. These included anxiety, depression, various psychotic states, abnormal smell and taste, dizziness, drowsiness, fatigue, confusion, headache, abnormal balance, difficulty in concentration, irritability, indecisiveness, and short-term memory loss (Murphy, 2014).

The disaster also caused social and economic problems. The area was already impoverished, and the disaster made the poverty worse. Family breadwinners had either died, and those who survived may have been physically harmed or emotionally traumatised permanently making a return to work, even when this was available, improbable. Young women who had been or were suspected of having been exposed to the gas suffered social stigma resulting in a diminution in their marriage prospects (Makwana, 2019).

Howard Duhon is a petrochemical engineer and was an employee of Union Carbide Corporation, the US parent company of the subsidiary in Bhopal at the time of the disaster. He states that he remembers exactly where he was when he first heard of the disaster at Bhopal. Decades later he travelled to Bhopal to see the site of the disaster and this is what he observed:

> Today, the accident is still alive in the neighborhood around the plant. Billboards and graffiti demand restitution. Hospitals and rehabilitation centers continue to treat the injured. Thousands still seek medical attention for problems, especially lung damage, and also immune system impairment, neurological damage, cancers, gynecological disorders, and mental health issues…
>
> (Duhon, 2014)

Much of the literature on what happened in Bhopal in 1984 uses the descriptive attribution of 'accident' as does Duhon. However, Duhon also shifts the perspective that it was an accident to an understanding that encompasses identifiable causes and responsibilities. Relying mainly on the analysis of the historical and cultural setting of the disaster by chemist and Union Carbide retiree Themistocles D'Silva (2006), he cites the continued negative effects of colonisation of India by the British (independence was gained in 1947), the overall poverty of the country and abject poverty in the Bhopal region including a shanty town around the plant, and the lack of safety measures generally in the country.

What Duhon also mentions is the tenor of the Indian legal system that undermined the ability of foreign companies to make a profit, and employee mistrust of management meaning when accidents did occur, they were not reported and therefore learning from mistakes was not possible, and claims that it is likely that the immediate cause was sabotage by a disgruntled employee. What is mentioned in a report by the human rights organisation Amnesty International (2004) is that the Union Carbide Bhopal plant had been polluting groundwater and soil since it began functioning in the early 1970s. Although abandoned after the disaster, groundwater continued to be polluted by remaining toxins in the plant 20 years later.

Primarily because of poor waste disposal practices. The plant site, abandoned since the 1984 leak, continues to pollute the groundwater, the sole source of water for those around the plant, with many toxic substances, that according to some reports may be carcinogenic. This has also resulted in thousands more people being poisoned. Despite knowledge about the extent of contamination and repeated entreaties to do so, Union Carbide has not taken substantive action to clean the plant site, and on the night of the gas leak crucial safety systems were not operating and safety concerns about the plant had previously been raised by auditors, the media, and the worker's union. There is in the Amnesty report (2004), however, the claim that both national and local Indian governing bodies had failed to comply with their obligations and responsibilities to prevent the gas leak and address their consequences.

Contagions and Mental Health

From the start of the COVID-19 pandemic and over the subsequent years there has been an outpouring of hypothesising and empirical evidence of varying size and quality assessing the state of mental health in particular groups. There has been judgement made on the mental health status of the old, the young, women, men, ethnic and social class groupings, people with a pre-existing mental disorder diagnosis, and those who are intellectually disabled, as well as whole populations including what of the whole world. Added to this mass of material on mental health and COVID-19 has been an abundance of postulating and investigation into physical health and COVID-19 and whether the disease affects morbidity and mortality rates in those people who were previously diagnosed with a mental disorder or were diagnosed during the years of the pandemic.

COVID-19 is cast as a disaster 'like no other disaster' for the momentous despoiling of the mind. For journalist Jacob Stern, COVID-19 is catastrophic for mental health and uniquely so:

> This Is Not a Normal Mental-Health Disaster…..the psychological effects of the novel coronavirus will long outlast the pandemic itself. [capitals in original]
>
> (Stern, 2020)

There has accrued a wealth of evidence from multiple sources linking high levels and abundant occurrences of mental unwellness to this pandemic. The evidence indicates that the mental health of both children and adults is detrimentally affected. Moreover, the COVID-19 pandemic is blamed for initiating or intensifying a wide range of psychological suffering across the world, some of which has been diagnosed as mental disorder, either in both those who have previously been infected by the virus and those who have not.

Examples of diagnosable psychological suffering commonly indicted include the following: anxiety (broad-spectrum, social, and specific states of angst such as germaphobia and claustrophobia); other forms of ontological unease due, for example, to fears of unemployment and destitution; psychosis; depression; loneliness; post-traumatic stress; bereavement/grief; compulsive-obsessiveness; insomnia; addictiveness (for example, to alcohol and online-shopping); aggression (notably against women); and various symptoms of psychosis such as hallucinations, delusions, and disordered thoughts (Taquet *et al.*, 2021; World Health Organisation, 2022a; Xie *et al.*, 2022).

It is not only people with a perceived mental health status that is different to the norm based on a diagnosis of mental disorder who have been identified as excessively susceptible to the ill effects of COVID-19. As is the case with those diagnosed with a mental disorder. In non-pandemic times people assessed formally as having an 'intellectual disability' are also vulnerable to dying earlier than the average age of death for the overall population. Exposure to COVID-19 exacerbates that difference (Das-Munshi *et al.*, 2021).

In 2020 representatives from The Royal College of Paediatrics and Child Health were reported by the BBC warning that the COVID-19 pandemic and resultant public health measures such as quarantine were major reasons for an increase in eating disorders in children and young people (Mundasad, 2020). Specifically, this increase was blamed on the separation from face-to-face contact with friends and from school activities, fears about contracting the disease, and mounting family worries about finances. The British National Health Service data collecting service conducted in July 2020 reported that 'probable' mental disorder had increased since 2017 (NHS Digital, 2020). Notably, the report stated that by 2020 the rate of mental disorder in children had (probably) risen from one in nine to one in six children in England aged 5 to 16 years. It is suggested in the report that these mental traumas may also contribute to brain traumas in the shape of cerebral inflammation, and neuro-immunological perturbation. In the same year that report was published further empirical evidence emerged indicating that serious mental disorder and noticeable changes in neurological functioning associated with COVID are interrelated (Mazza *et al.*, 2020; Patterson, *et al.*, 2020; Rogers *et al.*, 2020; Taquet *et al.*, 2021). There was also evidence that COVID-19 could detrimentally affect the elemental anatomy and physiology of the brain (Marshall, 2020). More and more data accrued in the following two years pointing in the same direction, that is, linking the disease to neurological pathology and very high levels of mental disorder.

The World Health Organisation (WHO, 2022a) observes that during the first year of the COVID-19 pandemic, the mental health of young people had worsened, and they became disproportionally at risk of suicide and self-harm. Moreover, women more than men, and those with pre-existing physical health conditions, such as asthma, cancer, and heart disease, were more likely to develop symptoms of mental disorders. Those people who have been particularly at risk of contracting severe physical suffering and dying from COVID-19 also included those already diagnosed with a mental disorder, especially young people diagnosed with psychosis.

In a study examining the mental health of staff working in intensive care units in English hospitals during COVID-19, the researchers concluded that there were substantial rates of (probable) mental health disorders and thoughts of self-harm especially prevalent in nurses (Greenberg *et al.*, 2021). What is noted by World Health Organisation (WHO, 2022a) is a rise in suicidal rumination among health workers during this first year of the pandemic. Health workers had faced the enormous challenge of dealing with seriously ill and dying patients without having enough appropriate protective equipment thereby making them susceptible to cross-infection. Health systems were also understaffed to deal with the huge influx of seriously ill patients, and this situation was made worse when staff *in situ* contracted COVID-19 and therefore had to stop working. Added to these problems was a lack of technical equipment such as respirators. In the circumstances, health workers became exhausted. Another study reported negative effects on the mental health of health and care workers in frontline roles during the COVID-19 pandemic. Psychological suffering was associated with fear of becoming infected and infecting others, not being able to cope with the increased workload, feeling stigmatised, and having insufficient access to effective personal protective equipment (Greene *et al.*, 2021). The correlatability of 'Long COVID', sequelae of COVID-19, with depression and anxiety have also been noted (Office of National Statistics, 2021).

During the height of the COVID-19[2] pandemic, many surveys were conducted and reported by the press on the mental health of whole populations and sections of a population. One such section was that of university students. For example, in late 2020 the BBC provided details of the results of a survey conducted by the UK National Union of Students in 2020. These results claimed to identify a high level of psychological suffering among university students:

> More than 50% of students say their mental health has declined since the Covid pandemic began, says a survey for the National Union of Students (NUS). Many of the 4,241 students surveyed in November [2020] say they have suffered stress, loneliness, anxiety and depression.
>
> (Johnson and Kendall, 2020)

In the BBC's account, National Union of Students President of the Larissa Kennedy National Union of Students is reported to have called upon governments to provide funding to support students.

Earlier in 2020 there had already been calls for action in the form of further evidence and preventative public health policy regarding direct, indirect, and intermingled psychological and social effects of the COVID-19 pandemic. Concern was being expressed in medical journals that social isolation, social distancing, and financial difficulties were increasing incidents of anxiety and depression especially in older adults and children, worsening already diagnosed mental illnesses (Holmes *et al.*, 2020). The media was also reporting the spread of fear amongst the public. The following account provided by 'Julie from Minnesota', who had two months previously contracted COVID-19, appeared in the British newspaper *The Guardian* in August 2020:

> I know it sounds crazy, and I don't know how to properly articulate it, but….it really felt like something was taking over my brain and my body.
>
> (Davis, 2020)

This article referred to the pre-print report of a study from Italy that identified a link between having suffered from COVID-19 and a host of diagnosable mental illnesses. The authors of study, which was published later that year (Mazza *et al.*, 2020), claimed that 'perturbation of the immune system' caused by the infection could, in turn, induce such neuro-pathologies as brain inflammation and, in turn, increase the risk of anxiety and depression. A high incidence of inflammation of the brain has been noted in other studies (see, for example, Patterson *et al.*, 2020). The suggestion that biological sequelae of COVID-19 can be the root of diagnosable mental illness is contrastable with the notion that psycho-social factors connected to COVID-19, such as fearfulness and loneliness, are primary instigators of subsequent and serious psychological suffering.

In large bold font, the only article covered on the front page of the British newspaper 'The i' in July 2021 was:

Police officers facing mental health crisis.

(Butterworth, 2021)

The article on that page then listed details of how three-quarters of 12,471 police officers reported in a poll conducted by the English and Welsh Police Federation having had 'mental health difficulties' due to the demands made on them during the COVID-19 pandemic. Further details of the poll were then offered on page 4 of the newspaper, supplemented by comments reported by the Chair of the Scottish Police Federation which accorded with the finding of this poll. Both sources, however, pointed to other factors than COVID-19 considered to be causing high levels of psychological suffering among police officers. These were referred to as 'heavy workloads' and 'increasing demands'. The article was repeated in the internet edition of the newspaper.

British royalty became involved in a public health campaign in England regarding psychological suffering during the COVID-19 pandemic. As part of the campaign, titled 'Every Mind Matters', the Duke and Duchess of Cambridge (who became The Prince and Princess of Wales when Queen Elizabeth 11 died in 2022) narrated film with the theme of encouraging the public to take care of their mental and physical well-being (Public Health England, 2020). The campaign, using data from the Office of National Statistics published in April 2020 made the following claim:

More than 4 in 5 (84.2%) Brits are worried about the effect that coronavirus is having on their life, with over half (53.1%) saying it was affecting their wellbeing and nearly half (46.9%) reporting high levels of anxiety.

(Public Health England, 2020)

What was offered in the campaign aimed at reducing the concerns of the British people is a series of 'NHS expert tips and advice'. These included keeping a regular routine and setting goals; getting good-quality sleep; regulating information uptake from social media and news broadcasts; engaging in pleasurable and novel activities; relaxing; eating healthily; and exercising. Undoubtedly, expert tips and advice have merit with regard to sustaining psychological stability in normal times but their impact during a contagion that infected hundreds of millions of people and killed millions did not diminish worry worldwide substantially. Worrying about COVID-19 had been and continues to be (or concern about the occurrence of a similar pandemic) rampant whether construed as diagnosable mental disorder.

Loneliness is not a mental disorder. But living alone and not having direct social contact with, for example, family members, friends, neighbours, and colleagues, can undermine mental health. A study by the market research company Ipsos MORI (2021) on behalf of the Royal Foundation of the (then) Duke and Duchess of Cambridge explored perceptions of parents in the UK had of the problems they faced during the early years of raising their children at the time of COVID-19 pandemic. The report indicated that parental loneliness had dramatically increased as parents had been considered cut off from face-to-face (interpersonal) social contact. The increase in loneliness for parents is reported as more apparent in the deprived areas. What is also mentioned, although not directly linked to loneliness, is that a significant minority of the parents considered that the pandemic would have a negative impact on their mental health.

Another example of commentary about loneliness connected to the COVID-19 pandemic appearing in the press was an article making the argument that loneliness is a more serious risk to health risk than smoking or obesity (Evans, 2021). Science writer and blogger Alice Gray is quoted in the article making the case that loneliness is already a widespread problem even prior to the pandemic. Gray suggests that loneliness has a negative effect on both physical health, including the brain and mental health. The brain being affected means maintaining psychological solidity is undermined further. A 'vitally needed' remedy for this effect argues Gray is social prescribing. Social prescribing means the prescribing by medical practitioners and other health practitioners of non-clinical activities such as gardening, dancing, social clubs, and art.

The conclusions from Harvard University's 'Making Caring Common Project' accord with the notion that there was already an epidemic of loneliness in the USA prior to the pandemic (Weissbourd *et al.*, 2021). However, the pandemic has increased the number of people experiencing loneliness. Data from the project indicate that more than a third of USA citizens faced 'serious loneliness' during the pandemic. Particularly vulnerable to loneliness and its negative effects are young adults and the mothers of young children. The report links loneliness to depression, anxiety, substance abuse, domestic abuse, heart disease, and early mortality.

Poorna Bell (2015) is an award-winning journalist and author who before the COVID-19 pandemic wrote about loneliness. She subsequently wrote about how the COVID-19 pandemic was affecting her and humanity, in general, when it was towards the end of a second year. Her comments that its detrimental effect on the 'core of who we are' was only then just beginning to be realised indicates that, in her opinion, the seriousness of the pandemic had not been taken seriously by individuals and governments.

There had been warnings for decades (and arguably there were indications from the time of the pneumonic and bubonic plagues) that an outbreak of a lethal infectious disease on the scale of an epidemic if not a pandemic was probable. Indeed, the warnings, from credible and multiple sources, were that an eruption of a deadly contagion, probably a 'spillover' from animals, was certain if preventative measures were not forthcoming, and in case prevention failed then preparation measures were made available.

Prevention would mean more prophylactic pharmaceuticals but significant societal shifts such as a major dislocation of animal-human contact, solving poverty and inequality, and the sorting out of food production and distribution to resolve impending widespread shortages and the social crises that would ensue. Preparation would mean more than personal protective equipment, but extensive supplies of curative medications, many of which would have to be newly developed and that would need significant financial and intellectual investment. Preparation also needs the immediate availability of masses of static and mobile medical facilities and teams of skilled personnel recruited anew so they would not deplete the numbers of staff needed to continue caring for non-pandemic ailments. To prevent a pandemic the societal shift needs to be global. Likewise, global preparation is necessary for a pandemic. These requirements are so sizeable and so expensive that it is understandable in political and economic terms why they have not been implemented. It is not acceptable in moral terms.

For Bell, however, the pandemic got personal. After contracting COVID-19 she then, at the time of her writing about the experience, had suffered from 'Long COVID' for ten months. Her commentary includes a reference to her anger about being ill. This anger seems in part because her social and budget plans have been disrupted. Bell also mentions how overindulgence in her use of social media increased her anxiety. More than anxiousness, what Bell is indicating is that her psychological stableness had been undermined. She refers to how she seems as if she is looking down a 'dark corridor', and that she has 'lost time'. She also writes about how not knowing what was going to happen next because events are beyond her control has generated a fear of 'things going wrong', 'cognitive dissonance', and 'mental paralysis'.

The deterioration in mental health during the COVD-19 pandemic appears to be attendant to specific 'stressors' that have been identified repeatedly. The research led by epidemiologist Michael Marmot *et al.* (2020) identifies financial difficulties possibly through loss of employment, loneliness, boredom, frustration, fear of becoming infected, trepidation about the future, and impediments to accessing goods and amenities including essential food products, and health, social care, and emergency services. Mental health deterioration may mean an increase in prevailing psychological suffering or new experiences of suffering psychologically. As have other researchers, periods of lockdown and social distancing are identified by Marmot and his colleagues to be particularly stressful. Along with other studies, the research by Marmot and his colleagues reveals these stressors increase the risk of a mental disorder diagnosis of, for example, anxiety, depression, and PTSD. What is also highlighted by Marmot and his colleagues is that the psychological suffering from the pandemic reduces job opportunities and worsens financial security and thereby increasing the risk of further mental health deterioration. There is the danger of creating an unstoppable double-helix spiral of social and psychological problems. This becomes all the more possible after a social crisis such as the COVID-19 pandemic because of wider societal (most likely global) economic and employment deteriorations. Contagions and conflicts, while beneficial for some – notably those selling weapons and medicines, and contracted to rebuild societal systems and structures), in the main can result in further crises in society, and they could ignite further psychological suffering.

Researchers from the University College London conducted a 'COVID-19 Social Study' that tracked for two years starting from March 2020 the psychological and social consequences of the COVID-19 pandemic in the UK. In their final report published in September 2022, the researchers provide their findings, discuss the use the UK Government made of the findings as they occurred during the two years and how policy changes affected people's daily lives, and they also make recommendations (Fancourt *et al.*, 2022). The study involved more than 70,000 participants who contributed 1.2 million questionnaires, and more than 400 in-depth qualitative interviews. Dissemination of the results has been widespread with more than 100 academic papers published, and dozens of keynote conference speeches made. The authors of the COVID-19 Social Study final report claim that data from the study became one of the most widely used social science resources relating to the pandemic for the making of public health policies. Consultations have been given to UK government departments, the World Health Organisation, and over 100 third-sector organisations.

What is noted in the final report of the COVID-19 Social Study final report is the availability of copious amounts of literature on social isolation and its effects on physical and psychological well-being. Some of the available literature covers social isolation as an upshot of pandemic events. This literature includes situations of enforced 'lockdowns' when pandemics strike. These lockdowns have taken the form of a legal requirement for everyone (except, for example, emergency workers and a few politicians) to stay indoors and not to have contact with anyone from outside the individual's household. This happened with the arrival and spread of SARS-CoV-1 and SARS-CoV-2. The enforced isolation was drastic and draconian and did not always have a legal standing when the various plagues struck and victims along with non-infected relatives, were literally 'locked' in their houses.

But the authors of the COVID-19 Social Study final report argue that the form of social isolation that occurred during this pandemic was special. They claim that the quarantine measures adopted during the COVID-19 pandemic shared only some similarities with previous wide-spreading infectious diseases. Oddly, however, the authors seem to be comparing the COVID-19 outbreak with previous 'epidemics' rather than pandemics. Perhaps more pertinent regarding what makes the COVID-19 pandemic different is how easily it spread globally due to the fast and profuse movement of people that characterises modern modes of living. Further pertinency arises from the realisation that what also spreads at speed and copiously are the social and psychological effects of COVID-19. The dynamic distribution of the disease suggests Fancourt and her colleagues, renders its effects uniquely unpredictable.

Other contemporary catastrophes may well display similar unpredictable cause-and-effect characteristics. Warfare today operates at speed using hi-tech weaponry and with copious amounts of armoury. However, the proposal that a particular contemporary contagion or conflict is capricious is counter-intuitive given the increasingly sophisticated and computerised investigatory and modelling technology, aided increasingly by artificial intelligence, is applied to eruptions of disease and violence.

The conclusions of the COVID-19 Social Study are first that the pandemic did indeed affect the UK population detrimentally both in terms of the degree of psychological suffering. The greater the intensity of the disease in terms of virulence and number of cases the worse became the population's mental health.

But, once more there is a paradox or at least an unexpected corollary concerning restrictions and lockdowns:

> Worsening mental health coincided with higher rates of COVID-19, tighter restrictions, and the weeks leading up to lockdowns. Mental health then generally improved during lockdowns and most people were able to adapt and manage their wellbeing.
>
> (Fancourt *et al.*, 2022, p.72)

But there is a major caveat to this trend. The researchers also found that a sizeable proportion of the population suffered psychologically disproportionately during lockdowns compared with the rest of people in the UK. This was the proportion of the population characterised by precursory vulnerabilities including low educational attainment, low income, living in overcrowded conditions, and psychological and physical debilitation. Lockdowns led to an intensification of these vulnerabilities.

Another conclusion from COVID-19 Social Study is that death rates escalated. This is, of course, expected when, at that time, a lethal disease has not been contained or abated having run its course. But what is unexpected is that this research revealed that both thinking about self-harm and carrying out acts of self-harm increased along with ruminating about dying.

There were also gender differences, with women (especially if pregnant) suffering psychologically more than men. The mental health of key workers and people suffering with 'Long COVID-19' also worsened during the pandemic. A further finding is that public trust in politicians in the UK was lost during the pandemic when reports appeared in the media some that the most senior political figures and their advisors did not follow the rules. Some of these powerful people were very politicians who had made the rules they broke regarding social isolation.

A further point made in the report is that the psychological and social consequences of the pandemic will not stop when the disease abates. For example, the psychological aftereffects of personal financial loss and from losing a loved one, and the aftereffects on society from the pressure put on health services and the downturn in commercial activity, continue after any pandemic and most other types of disaster. Not all repercussions, however, are negative. The tenor of the final COVID-19 Social Study Final Report is that the repercussions of the pandemic are not only inevitable but are in the main harmful to people and society.

Moreover, the aftermath of the pandemic according to the report will add to prevailing global problems, and refer to political unrest, changes to the climate, and with specific reference to the UK, 'Brexit' (that is, the UK leaving the European Union which coincided with the start of the COVID-19 pandemic).

Regarding Brexit and mental health, there were accounts of psychological suffering appearing before the UK left the European Union but after the referendum had been conducted in 2016. According to a survey by the Mental Health Foundation Scotland conducted in the intervening years, almost two million adult Scots felt 'powerless', 'worried', and 'angry' due to Brexit before the exit. The adult population at that time was under 4.5 million. Adding to Scottish angst were experiences of interpersonal conflict involving family and friends over Brexit voting preferences. But, almost as an inconsequential aside, what is also recognised in the survey is that most people appeared to be coping, with a sizeable minority of Scots participating in the survey testifying that Brexit had affected them at all emotionally.

A study of survivors from the outbreak of the 2003 severe acute respiratory syndrome (SARS-CoV-1 to that of COVID-19 (SARS-CoV-2), including health workers, compared those in a control group. After a year the survivors still had higher levels of stress/anxiety, depression, anxiety, and post-traumatic symptoms, and scored higher in the General Health Questionnaire (a self-administered screening tool) indicating continued psychological suffering (Lee *et al.*, 2007).

Severe acute respiratory syndrome (SARS-CoV-1 and SARS-CoV-2) is a viral respiratory disease caused by a coronavirus. Coronaviruses are a large collection of viruses that infect humans and animals. Apart from SARS-CoV-1 and SARS-CoV-2, this group includes the common cold, and Middle East respiratory syndrome (MERS-CoV). Although the World Health Organisation (2023) states the first outbreak occurred in China early in 2003, the first case of SARS-CoV-1 has been identified retrospectively as occurring in November 2002 in the Guangdong province of China (Popescu, 2022). It then spread to more than two dozen countries in other parts of Asia, North America, South America, and Europe. Since containment occurred only eight months after the disease was first identified in 2003, only one outbreak has been reported. This was in April of the following year in China resulting from laboratory-acquired infection Centers for Disease Control and Prevention (2013).

Coronaviruses are dangerous because they spread easily through small droplets of saliva passing person-to-person via the respiratory system either directly through coughing or sneezing or indirectly by touching infected material including surfaces. The case fatality rate of those infected by SARS-CoV-1 and SARS-Cov-2 has been notoriously difficult to determine precisely. Assessing accurately the number of deaths is also problematic due to the way fatalities are recorded. In some countries, numbers are inefficiently collected, if collected then not declared publicly, or simply not collected. However, a figure of between 700 and 800 deaths from SARS-CoV-1 is agreed generally. Although each death is a tragedy, not least because a life is lost but also because of the negative consequences for the physical and mental health of secondary victims, the number of deaths from SARS-CoV-1 in comparison to those from SARS-CoV-2 is modest.

This has been attributed by the World Health Organisation (2023) to its own co-ordinating of the international investigation and response, helped by the Global Outbreak Alert and Response Network (GOARN), and health authorities in affected countries. Epidemiological data and clinical and logistical support, affirms the World Health Organisation, brought the outbreak under control. The Global Outbreak Alert and Response Network is also coordinated by the World Health Organisation, is an overarching agency that links hundreds of partners comprised of governments, the United Nations, and university and research institutions dealing with public health. Other partners are non-governmental organisations such as the International Committee of the Red Cross and Red Crescent Societies, *Médecins sans Frontières*, and the International Rescue Committee. The declared aim of the Global Outbreak Alert and Response Network is to prevent and control infectious disease outbreaks and public health emergencies when requested (World Health Organisation, 2015). The obvious question is, if such measures were implemented so competently for the SARS-CoV-1 outbreak, then why did the SARS-CoV-2 outbreak end up infecting billions and killing millions?

Long-term levels of diagnosable PTSD and depressive disorders reported amongst survivors of SARS-CoV-1 have been so high that it is suggested the outbreak furnished a 'mental health catastrophe':

[T]he SARS outbreak in 2003 should not simply be regarded as a medical event but also as a mental health catastrophe with a response compatible to that of other major disasters.

(Mak *et al.*, 2009, p.22)

However, psychiatrist Robert Maunder (2009) questions whether SARS-CoV-1 was really a mental health catastrophe. He accedes that these levels are consistent with previous studies that have reported persistent psychological symptoms amongst about half of the survivors of SARS-CoV-1 survivors, although the previous studies were not designed to diagnose psychiatric illnesses. But he argues these results need to be taken in the context of expected responses to other kinds of disasters.

After reviewing the literature on the effects of disasters on mental health, Maunder concludes that there is much evidence of the significantly raised prevalence of PTSD among direct victims of and, although to a lower level amongst rescue workers, compared to its occurrence in the general population. The evidence from the study by Mak and his colleagues, reflects Maunder, finds that following SARS-CoV-1 the prevalence of PTSD either higher or lower than it is found in other disasters. This discrepancy continues Maunder, depending on how the numbers of PTSD sufferers are counted. That is, in some studies all cases are counted whereas in others they are only counted if PTSD remains diagnosable at 30 weeks. If the latter method is adopted, points out Maunder, then nearly half of those who had suffered from PTSD after contracting SARS-CoV-1 had recovered from both. What Maunder misses, however, is that PTSD, and virtually all psychiatric classifications, are exposed to diagnostic uncertainty. Furthermore, Maunder does not reflect on the abiding and at times bitter debates about assigning medical labels to psychological suffering let alone emotions, behaviours, and thoughts that otherwise are classified as within the normal (or at least acceptable) spectrum of human performance.

There is nuance to Maunder's view that SARS-CoV-1 was not a mental health catastrophe. He clarifies that that the impact in terms of stress of infectious disease could be qualitatively distinct from that of other disasters. Infectious disease, especially if potentially lethal, has been from the times of the plague, managed through a policy of isolation even when this stratagem has been utilised out of raw panic rather than sound knowledge about pathogenic microorganisms and their modes of contamination. Today, the enactment by the State of sophisticated surveillance techniques and technologies, the use of personal protective equipment by health care professionals, and the widespread awareness of the dangers of contagious disease add to the stress placed on the population generally and, in particular, those who contract the disease. Added to the stress on sufferers is the social stigma associated with being infected which can continue after recovery. Furthermore, the infected individual may agonise about their own health and of infecting others, above all of passing the disease to vulnerable loved ones such as young offspring, elderly relatives, and any family member with a compromised immune system. This is likely to be of heightened concern for healthcare professionals dealing directly with infected patients.

Prompt containment of the SARS-CoV-1 outbreak was possible primarily, suggests Maunder, because within a few months primarily because of the size of the coronavirus means it is not liable to produce viable mutations, and those infected do not shed the virus before becoming symptomatic and therefore they can be isolated soon after they are identified being infected. SARS-CoV-1 is not a highly infectious disease and had it been, reasons Maunder this outbreak 'would have been a very different story'. Moreover, Maunder argues, because the human cost of the SARS-CoV-1 outbreak was not great, it was not a mental health catastrophe. Maunder then, prophetically, warns:

> It was perhaps a dress rehearsal for the catastrophe that could emerge with the long-overdue influenza pandemic or some similar emergent infectious disease, if we are not better prepared next time.
>
> (Maunder, 2009, p.316)

Maunder expands on his warning, declaring bluntly and unambiguously awareness of the psychological suffering caused by the dramatic outbreak of SARS-CoV-1 means that there must be preparation for future dramas from infectious diseases. That preparation should focus on building up the resilience of healthcare professionals and healthcare organisations to mitigate the damage to and destruction of life and mental well-being. What he could have added is the need to diminish the damage and destruction of elements key to the functioning of society from pandemics alongside of those related to healthcare that can lead to the undermining of physical and mental health.

Maunder mentions influenza in the context of building resilience prior to another emerging infectious disease but one that could prove far more dramatic than SARS-CoV-1. What was a very different story was the dramatic outbreak not of influenza (although that nearly happened in 2022) but SARS-CoV-2. That was a human catastrophe because the warnings were not heeded, and the drama of large-scale suffering ensued.

The United Nations in May of 2020 in a policy briefing declared that the mental well-being of whole populations was being affected negatively by the COVID-19 crisis and consequently, the well-being of whole societies was being affected negatively:

> Although the COVID-19 crisis is, in the first instance, a physical health crisis, it has the seeds of a major mental health crisis as well, if action is not taken. Good mental health is critical to the functioning of society at the best of times.
>
> (United Nations, 2020, p.2)

Even before the COVID-19 pandemic depression and anxiety not only affects hundreds of millions of people worldwide, but it is also calculated to cost the global economy annually more than US$1 trillion (United Nations, 2020). Therefore, argued the United Nations, preventing further costs to people and their communities must be a policy priority. The policy priorities to minimise the adverse impact on mental health from the pandemic recommended by the United Nations at that stage were threefold: (1) a whole-of-society approach to promote, protect and care for mental health; (2) widespread availability of emergency mental health support; (3) the building of better mental health services to enable recovery. But mitigation through a whole-of-society approach, making available emergency mental health support, and having available suitable mental health services to aid recovery, should have been policy priorities long before the arrival of SARS-CoV-2. There was no shortage of warnings that an emerging infectious disease would cause a pandemic was probable – and warnings are in place regarding future pandemics.

Primary accounts of the mental health of the populations affected by medieval and 17th-century plagues are limited. This is because most of the people, certainly at the time of the medieval waves of plague, were not literate, and if those who could write did document their experiences these documents have not endured. Another reason is likely to be that most people when faced with such a terrible disease are desperate to endure rather than desperate to ensure that their desperation is documented.

But one expansive first-hand source from which the state of the population's mental health not only in London but throughout Europe can be inferred is Daniel Defoe's journal (although written years after the event, and with added literary embellishment). In Defoe's journal, there are indications that there was a dramatic shift in attitudes, feelings, and behaviours towards outsiders with a desire for protection against those perceived to have brought the plague with them from foreign lands. The latter included both other European and non-European countries. The change in mindset was at the level of extreme fearfulness, paranoia, and despondency. Not only did the widescale number of deaths caused by the plague detrimentally affect the functioning of society but resulted in the substantial deterioration in the mental health of the survivors and which further undermined the ability of societal systems to recover (Masterpasqua and Perna, 1997).

The weight of evidence from contemporary times is supportive of the premise that contagions such as the coronaviruses that source serious acute respiratory syndromes have the effect of causing psychological suffering. It certainly can be claimed 'factually' that certain microorganisms cause certain diseases. But conclusions linking specific contagions to specific forms of psychological suffering (let alone specific mental disorders) can only be tentative. Most of the studies mentioned here implicitly or explicitly acknowledge that there is a 'probable' cause-and-effect relationship between these two variables rather than this being a fact.

Conflicts and Mental Health

The International Panel on Climate Change (IPCC) is an agency of the United Nations. The relationship between psychological suffering and the fear and experience of **climatic change** and catastrophe has been noted previously by the IPCC. In a 2022 report, there is much more detail about the risks to mental health from rising temperatures. The report is unequivocal, that the climate crisis is causing misfortune and misery to people and nature. The earth's ecology, animals, and humans, and moving towards not being able to adapt. Already 3.3 billion people live in highly vulnerable situations.

Emotional distress is linked to the worry about and from enduring, for example, flooding, drought, heat waves, fires, hurricanes, and cyclones. Diagnosable mental disorders such as generalised anxiety, depression, PSTD, and complex psychopathology (that is a mixture of mental disorders occurring simultaneously) can be triggered and pre-existing diagnosed mental disorders can worsen, due to these events. A rise in rates of admissions to psychiatric in-patient facilities, violence and suicide, can also be the eventual consequences of escalating temperatures and sea levels.

There has also been a specific term conceived to describe the emotional distress connected to the climate emergency, 'solastalgia':

> As opposed to nostalgia – the melancholia or homesickness experienced by individuals when separated from a loved home – solastalgia is the distress that is produced by environmental change.
>
> (Albrecht *et al.*, 2007, p.S95)

This form of psychological suffering is associated with the loss of or damage to homes, land, local amenities, employment opportunities, community connectedness, and displacement, when, for example, floods or fires strike. Displacement may result when an area is severely damaged or destroyed either through armed conflict or climatic conflict. Each year since 2008 more than 20 million people have been displaced within their own countries by weather-related extreme events (IPCC, 2022). Individuals and families may find themselves amongst stranger populations in overcrowded and unsanitary conditions, thereby contributing further to their emotional distress. There are also multiple risks to physical health when displaced into situations that can be inadequate in terms of shelter, ventilation, the regular supply of clean water, sanitation, and access to health care including immunisation. These risks include malnutrition, and greater vulnerability to infection from cholera, dysentery, typhoid fever, hepatitis, measles, meningitis, and acute respiratory infection, malaria, dengue, and sexually transmitted diseases (McMichael *et al.*, 2012).

There is caution in the IPCC report, however, about such terms as solastalgia and leaping to causative relationships between the climate emergency, worrying about this, and diagnosable mental disorder. Also, data on such relationships is also missing from large parts of the world (for example, in Africa, South and Central America, and Asia) and where mental disorder as well as suicide, is stigmatised and therefore may not be recorded officially.

The IPCC recommend adaptation options for reducing the mental health risks associated with the climate crisis. These include improving the monitoring of populations affected directly by climatic shifts, access to mental health care. To assist survival the IPCC suggests improvements in the integration and governance of policies and practices of the societal structures and systems supporting and supplying health care, water and food, sanitation, and livelihoods.

Research by social policy scholar Caroline Hickman and her colleagues (Hickman *et al.*, 2021) involved surveying the views of 10,000 children and young people regarding their thoughts and feelings about the climate crisis, and how governments were responding to the crisis. These researchers regard climate anxiety (and by implication also eco anxiety) as complex as well as understandable.

> Although painful and distressing, climate anxiety is rational and does not imply mental illness. Anxiety is an emotion that alerts us to danger...However, because the climate crisis is so complex and lacks a clear solution, anxiety can easily become too intense and even overwhelming.
>
> (Hickman *et al.*, 2021, p.e863)

It can instil many psychological responses including anger, grief, and despair. Other reactions include feelings of shame and guilt about not taking personal responsibility and action to alter the climatic and ecological conditions that have led to these crises. Conversely, hopefulness can be engendered whereby there is a belief that solutions can be found that ally or possibly reverse the harm done to the climate, the environment, and biodiversity.

New descriptors of the psychological suffering attributed to climate change other than climate anxiety, ecoanxiety, and solastalgia (Cianconi *et al.*, 2020). Examples include ecoguilt and ecological grief. New academic specialities and interdisciplinary groupings have also been established and others revitalised as a consequence of the climate crisis. These include climate psychology, ecopsychology, ecopsychiatry, the climate psychiatry alliance, ecosociology, environmental sociology, and ecological anthropology, as well as the various subdivisions of neuroscience engaged in investigating how the effects of the climate emergency may affect the brain and other neurological tissues and organs. The research from these disciplines covers the psychological and biological upshots on individuals and populations from both worrying about what might happen and what has already happened.

The effects on human performance of social crises such as climatic disasters can be direct or indirect, short-term, or long-term. Behavioural, cognitive, and emotional alterations may be immediate, delayed, short-lasting, or long-lasting (Cianconi *et al.*, 2020). Both contagions and conflicts (including humanity's disastrous conflict with nature) cause alterations in human performance. Some of these changes are necessarily major. To survive life-threatening situations such as contamination from a deadly disease such as Ebola, or the impending arrival of a tsunami, people need to urgently separate themselves or wear full protective equipment such as a hazmat suit, or instantly find ground at a higher level than the approaching waves. The loss of life and property from the inundation of giant waves can produce delayed but nevertheless severe effects, notably PTSD. Moreover, social crises can affect different populations in different ways (Cianconi *et al.*, 2020). People living in impoverished parts of the world, in areas of low land, and those who do not have the material, informational, and psychological resources, and societal infrastructures to enable recovery.

For psychologist Susan Clayton (2021) the expanding number of studies demonstrating that not only can extreme weather events associated with the climate crisis affect mental health negatively, and increase the diagnoses of anxiety, depression, and PTSD, in particular, but more gradual changes to the climate can also accentuate psychological suffering. She cites the example of ambient environmental conditions worsening leading to a reduction in the quality of air and heightened temperatures. She also notes that both dramatic and modest consequences of the climate crisis do not affect all groups equally. The social context matters. As already noted, not only are some countries and some regions within counties such as low-lying areas, the poor, and those without access to resources, vulnerable, but women are disproportionate to men, children, indigenous populations, as well as people with pre-existing diagnoses of mental disorder.

Clayton points to a paradox (yes, yet another one).[3] Social networks, remarks Clayton, can exaggerate or minimise the perceived threat of the climate crisis (that is, increase or decrease a reaction that may cause worry about whether this could be classified as 'climate anxiety' or 'ecoanxiety'). Ironically, however, people who belong to social networks that are well-informed about the climate crisis, and this could apply to any other disaster, may experience worse worry than those who are either un-informed or have succumbed to denial. The deniers may merely have effective mental defence mechanisms protecting them from worrying about or climate crisis or any of life's other vicissitudes, or because they believe conspiracy propaganda that it is in the interests of the politically and commercially powerful to divert attention from their disempowered plight or to sell them commodities aimed at protecting them from a disaster that will never occur. Denial, argues Clayton, only works in the short term to lower worry. Ultimately, whatever is the (real) crisis, while denial about its causes may remain, its effects will be unavoidable. This includes the effect on mental health. A further irony applies to the well-informed. They may be able to call upon their social networks to provide support and assets to help them adapt to the environmental, physical, and psychological consequences of crises.

Research by the British Association for Counselling and Psychotherapy on the impact of the climate emergency on mental health concluded that ecoanxiety affects more than half of adults in the UK. The nub of the anxiety for the participants in the study is a sense of powerlessness, a feeling that their ability to partake in effective means to reduce the possibility of ecological catastrophe is limited or absent. What the researchers conducting this study also report is that participants expressed 'genuine anxiety and depression' for themselves, future generations, and the planet. Concern was also conveyed about disadvantaged people because, in the view of the participants, are more vulnerable to the consequences of the climate emergency.

In an interesting twist in psychological terms, however, the researchers point out that not responding anxiously to an impending disaster replete with devastating floods, fires, famine, and fighting, would signify dysfunction. That is, it is highly appropriate to be worried and despondent about catastrophe. Ecoanxiety therefore in these circumstances is not a pathological emotion but a rational response. Furthermore, ecoanxiety may be a functional aspect of human performance that does empower people and lead to changes that then lead to diminishing the threat of ecocide and the demise of humanity. From this perspective for those experiencing ecoanxiety the remedies of psychiatrists, psychologists, or psychotherapists would be counterproductive. There is a perspective that regards interventions from these professionals are counterproductive or even destructive for much psychological suffering. Suffering may be an integral and indispensable element of human existence, enabling not disabling future psychological solidity to the extent that personal growth becomes more feasible (Morrall, 2017).

Adrian James, President of the Royal College of Psychiatrists has commented on how environmental conditions impact mental health both negatively and positively:

> The environmental and climate emergency is also a mental health emergency. Our health is fundamentally linked to the quality of our environment, whether that's about cleaner air, access to green spaces or protection from extreme weather.
> (James quoted in King's College London News, 2021)

The World Health Organisation (2022b) calculates that globally more than 55 million people suffer from dementia. Dementia is a wide-ranging syndrome characterised by cognitive decline linked to the deterioration of physical brain matter more than expected as part of the normal ageing process. According to a report examining the connection between air pollution and dementia by the UK Government's Committee on the Medical Effects of Air Pollutants (2022), one-fifth of people over the age of 65 years in England is estimated to be mildly cognitively impaired. Up to 10% of those already experiencing cognitive impairment will eventually develop dementia. It is one of the leading causes of death from disease, and a major cause of disability and dependency (World Health Organisation, 2022b).

Alongside the psychological and social challenges dementia poses for the sufferer and her/his family, it is one of the greatest challenges to society because of the need for providing substantially more health and social care than is offered presently because the population of many Western countries is ageing. But it is not confined to the elderly. Nor might the causative factors be confined to those directly to do with the individual's biology or personally controllable lifestyle. High blood pressure and smoking are accepted causative culprits. But societal and environmental factors are also suspected of making dementia more likely.

There is mounting epidemiological evidence that air pollution may contribute to both the decline in cognitive function and to the development of dementia (Committee on the Medical Effects of Air Pollutants, 2022). Small particle pollutants in the atmosphere are the most dangerous to health. They are known to contribute to heart and lung disease. It is the damage done to these physiological systems connecting the heart and lungs, especially to blood vessels, that is suspected of causing 'vascular' dementia. The immune system may also be involved. Immune cells may be released in the brain when provoked by these foreign particles. In the ensuing combat between these otherwise protective cells and the interlopers, brain tissue is damaged. Sources of the fine particles that undermine health include the exhausts of combustion engine vehicles, smoke from the burning of wood, oil, coal, and forest and grass fires, and the gases and droplets released emitted from industrial vents including those in power plants. Fine particles accumulate where there is heavy and slow-moving traffic, and where there is little wind to disperse fumes from fires and industry. As yet, it is not clear which from a long list of possible particles, are those that are the most harmful to cerebral well-being.

Apart from dementia, exposure to traffic-related air pollution may be a factor responsible for increasing the likelihood of a diagnosis of a serious mental disorder, and of worsening the mental health in those already diagnosed with schizophrenia, bipolar disorder, and depression. In a study conducted in 2019 measuring the use of mental health services in areas of London of dense traffic and residents it was found that in-patient numbers increased as did the requirement for community support (Newbury *et al.*, 2021). The study's authors argue for the reduction of air pollution to be adopted as an important 'population-level' policy aimed at improving the course of psychotic and mood disorders. Improving air quality can improve mental health or at least not add to existing psychological suffering. Air pollution, however, is just one of many of society's insanities that if conciliated would work to improve mental health far more effectively than placatory pharmaceuticals or psychotherapies aimed at individuals.

Pollution leads to ecocide. To be clear, ecocide means severe and longlasting damage and destruction of ecosystems. It does not necessarily mean that all life forms are obliterated. Some forms of life may hang on no matter how cataclysmic an episode of ecocide. Extraneous plants and/or animals may re-populate the area of destruction, taking advantage of the absence of competitors. The lineage of life is replete with episodes of obliteration and regeneration. One example of this process occurred 250 million years ago, at the end of the Permian historical epoch when a mass extinction ended nearly all of life on earth. The end-Permian extinction occurred in stages, each one epitomising Armageddon. This was all taking place in a single land mass that came to be called Pangea. Pangea was a combination of what fragmented during the Triassic epoch eventually forming, in approximate terms, the continents of North America, South America, Africa, and Europe.

The atmosphere was already depleted of oxygen before the first of two occurrences of colossal volcanic explosions. This was due to hot climatic conditions drying much of the land making oxygen-releasing life (plants) scarcer and breathing for animals severely impaired. In the first, a plume of magma erupted from deep within the earth in what is now China. Lava and noxious gasses created a massive hike in the greenhouse effect, acidified the oceans, and destroyed much of the ozone layer. A few million years after that catastrophe, another occurred in what is now Siberia. Another magma eruption, but this time much larger than its predecessor and thereby far more toxic. The lava and gasses from this second event were much more devastating to life on earth than the first, nearly bringing all of it to an end over a period of half-a-million years. Palaeontologist, and evolutionary biologist Henry Gee (2021) describes how 19 out of 20 species of animal in the sea and seven out of every ten in this Hell-on-earth were poisoned, asphyxiated, burned, boiled, broiled, fried, or dissolved. The planet was left bare, silent, and dying.

But of course, life returned. It is possible, although not recommended as a policy, that a failure to prevent the present day move towards another climatic Armageddon will annihilate most life and that other species will repopulate the earth and a species other than humans will dominate.

A report in 2006 by the international environment campaigning organisation Greenpeace on the effects of the 1986 Chernobyl Catastrophe on health states unambiguously that serious illness is connectable to the radioactivity released from the release of radioactivity at the power plant:

> Today it is clear that the pollution from Chernobyl has indeed caused a largescale increase in cancers.....
>
> (Greenpeace, 2006, p.11)

Greenpeace cites the higher prevalence of kidney, urinary/bladder, and thyroid cancer in the liquidators from Belarus, for the period from 1993 to 2003 than what they refer to as 'comparable reference group'. Leukaemia, for Greenpeace, was also significantly higher in liquidators from Ukraine, as well as in adults in Belarus and in children in the most contaminated areas of Ukraine and Russia. There has been amongst the affected population, argues Greenpeace, increased morbidity from diseases of the respiratory, digestive, vascular, muscular-skeletal immune, reproductive, and urinary-genital systems, and of genetic abnormalities. Greenpeace, posits that the Intelligence Quotient of some of the 'Chernobyl Children' is lower than in a control group, and neurological and psychiatric disorders are at a higher rate in adults than expected levels. The latter include depression, anxiety, and PTSD, and unexplained somatisation symptoms. A comparison is drawn between the Chernobyl catastrophe and the exposure of

Japanese populations when atomic bombs hit Nagasaki and Hiroshima in August of 1945. Greenpeace notes that many of the survivors were still experiencing symptoms of anxiety and somatisation, and the diagnosis of schizophrenia was 'very high', decades after the bombings.

There continues to be disagreement about both the final morbidity and mortality toll from the 1986 Chernobyl disaster. Direct deaths are counted in the tens but those and others who have died indirectly from the effects of the disaster could be in the tens of thousands (Longmuir and Agyapon 2022). Unforeseen contamination has come from inadvertent sources. For example, at the same time as when people were being evacuated from the area around Chernobyl, thousands of animals were slaughtered. Some of the fleeces of these animals, along with more contaminated wool from northern Ukrainian farms covered in radioactive clouds from the explosion, seem to have ended up in a factory in a town about 85 kilometres from Chernobyl (Gray, 2019).

Radioactive iodine is linked to thyroid cancer, Strontium to leukaemia, and Caesium can detrimentally impact on the whole body and is especially harmful to the liver and spleen. According to the International Atomic Energy Agency (2023), the disaster at the Chernobyl power plant in 1986, 1,800 cases of thyroid cancer in children have been documented. The thyroid is an endocrine gland produces hormones necessary for the regulation of the body's metabolic rate. The metabolic rate influences the functioning of core organs including the heart and the brain. Unfortunately, the thyroid gland is susceptible to absorbing certain radioactive materials such as the iodine released from the Chernobyl explosion. Young children are especially vulnerable to radioactive iodine uptake. Regarding adults, the International Atomic Energy Agency reports that there is no solid evidence that the radioactive release from Chernobyl caused cancer or disease.

But there is evidence of the cost to the mental health of those working at Chernobyl and the people living in the surrounding areas of the Chernobyl power plant, and the liquidators (the liquidators were the emergency workers drafted in to clean up the plant premises and the surrounding area):

> The psychological affects [sic] of Chernobyl were and remain widespread and profound, and have resulted for instance in suicides, drinking problems and apathy.
>
> (International Atomic Energy Agency, 2023)

There is evidence of harm done from radioactivity to nature and to animal populations. For example, mutations and deformities did occur in plants and animals after the plant explosion. Leaves changed shape and some animals were born with physical deformities. But notwithstanding persistently higher levels of radiation in the parts of the originally affected area, there is regrowth of vegetation. Animals, including beavers, moose, wolves, wild boar, and multiple bird species, have returned and seem to be thriving. Some former residents have gone back willingly to their homes. Moreover, prior to the 2022 invasion of Ukraine by Russia, Chernobyl attracted tourism (International Atomic Energy Agency, 2023).

While there is controversy about how many people have died from the catastrophe at Chernobyl there is little disagreement that nuclear 'accidents', and warfare result in psychological suffering. Moreover, there is mentioned in the literature the diagnosis of particular mental disorders following actual nuclear disasters (both accidents and warfare) and from the fear of such events. Especially exposed to psychological suffering are those who are especially exposed to radiation fallout. They are people living and working near the nuclear facility, the emergency personnel and the decontamination workforce sent to deal with the aftermath, and evacuees. As with the Chernobyl, the Three Mile Island and the Fukushima nuclear disasters are associated with higher levels of depression, and anxiety, and PTSD (Longmuir and Agyapon, 2022).

Radiation anxiety is cognitive negativity induced by a fear of contamination and its effects. It can be defined as follows:

> [A]nxiety due to perceived radiation exposure, actual radiation exposure, or potential for radiation exposure in the future… [including] concern about current health status, delayed health effects, and genetic effects on offspring and future generations.
>
> (Longmuir and Agyapon, 2022)

Comparable to the Chernobyl catastrophe, increased incidents of symptoms and potential diagnosis of anxiety, depression, PTSD, as well as alcohol abuse and suicide, are associated with the Fukushima Daiichi disaster. But connecting causally the predictable and comprehensible worry about the risk of radiation contamination with either symptoms or a full diagnosis of a mental disorder is problematic. There is not necessarily a linear causal pathway between worry and mental disorder. Many social and psychological characteristics of communities and individuals intervene to avert, distort, or augment, that linkage. Moreover, there is substantial residual resilience in catastrophic situations including nuclear events that can protect from debilitating emotional distress in the short-term and long-term. Carefully selected psycho-social interventions by the State, local authorities, and professionals, can assist in sustaining and enhancing resilience (Kobayashi *et al.*, 2022).

Apart from those who died immediately when in August 1945 the USA dropped atomic bombs on the Japanese cities of Hiroshima and Nagasaki, many more died soon after the explosions because of a breakdown in the rescue and medical services and the absence of personnel (many of whom were also dead or dying) to operate those services. Those people who had not been killed but who were in the general vicinity of the explosions suffered the agonising effects of radiation. Katharine Hudson is the General Secretary of the Campaign for Nuclear Disarmament. She describes what happened in vivid detail what happened in Hiroshima. She explains how the core of the explosion reached a temperature of several million degrees centigrade was reached in the core of the explosion. This resulted in a flash of heat that killed every person within half a mile, vapouring their bodies. Their death rate wasn't much less further away when the continuing heat and then shock waves, falling debris, and fires, killed over 90% of the people and destroyed or damaged about the same percentage of buildings. Those left alive were still vulnerable:

> Within two or three days, radiation victims who were near the hypo-centre developed symptoms such as nausea, vomiting, bloody diarrhoea and hair loss. Most died within a week. Radiation victims further away from the explosion developed symptoms one to four weeks after the explosion.
>
> (Hudson, 2013)

After a few years, a higher rate of cancer became evident. These cancers were of the thyroid, breasts, lungs, and salivary glands. Hudson goes on to describe the horror of what happened to the women who were pregnant and had survived. Many of their babies were stillborn, and if born may not have lived long. Some of those children who did live longer did so with severe physical abnormalities and/or severe distress emotionally.

Given what happens to disturb mental health when there is a nuclear accident it might be expected that a nuclear attack would spawn severe and long-lasting psychological suffering among many if not most of the survivors. Aside from the physical harm from radiation, affecting survivors (some of whom would later die from the effects of radiation) a higher prevalence of anxiety symptoms and somatisation symptoms (that is the expression of physical symptoms which are probably psychological in origin such pain and fatigue) was found in a study examining the mental health of survivors from **Hiroshima and Nagasaki** 20 years after the dropping of the bombs (Yamada and Izumi, 2002). A study of survivors 50 years after the bombing of Nagasaki, however, revealed surprising results. Compared to a control group, unspecific emotional distress was greater in the survivors as were indications of difficulty in activities of everyday living (for example, in maintaining relationships, enjoyment in and enthusiasm for their lives). Emotional distress was more profound amongst survivors who were still ruminating about their experience of having a nuclear bomb dropped on their city. But there were fewer indications of anxiety and depression among the survivors compared with those in the control group (Ohta *et al.*, 2000).

It would seem extremely sensible and exceptionally insensitive not to accept that there would be considerable harm to mental health after enduring the horrors of genocide. The Holocaust is probably perhaps humanity's most horrific genocidal event. Clinical and academic commentary of Holocaust survivors continues to underscore that ostensibly patent perspective on serious psychological suffering from this exceptionally extreme genocidal episode:

> The Holocaust was one of the most traumatic catastrophes in recorded human history. Survivors seeking psychotherapeutic help today, now in their seventies and older, often show symptoms of a posttraumatic stress disorder (PTSD), depression, or prolonged grief disorder.
>
> (Forstmeier *et al.*, 2020)

In the years after they left the concentration camps, psychiatrists began describing the psychological suffering of the survivors who were not surviving psychologically as 'survivor syndrome' and 'concentration camp syndrome'. These novel diagnoses were in the main to be subsumed under the psychiatric category of PTSD. Psychiatrists were not the only professionals concerned with the suffering of the Holocaust survivors. Psychoanalytic psychotherapists come to the forefront of the professionalised management of survivors' mental health (LaCapra, 2001). The non-professionalised input of families and agencies, including religious organisations offering support and the establishment of the State of Israel, as well as the spirit of the survivors were just as vital, if not more so, than that of trauma specialists, in their emotional struggles in the aftermath of the Holocaust (Hass, 1995).

For historian Arthur Marwick (1988), wars, not even ones that engage a multitude of countries and encompass multiple continents if not the world in totality, are not independent factors disengaged from a plethora of societal inclinations that may have been a long time gestating and may have set the scene for what seems sudden change. Wars, particularly 'total wars', are significant catalysts for social change but protracted historical trends are the roots of shifts in the direction of a society's culture, economics, and politics. These shifts in society, notes Marwick, can be either progressive or regressive. The condition of society, whether stable or unstable and the human psyche, whether suffering or solid, are inexorably interlinked.

War offers the opportunity to concoct a variant of the law of unintended consequences, the law of unacknowledged but inevitable consequences. The intense excitement felt by prospective combatants on the expectation of new experiences and of engaging in what may be presented as a praiseworthy and purposeful pursuit by governmental propagandists or idealistic activists, and the practical payoffs from increased employment opportunities arising from increased production of how to conduct warfare, belie what will subsequently be realised are the terrible realities of warfare. The scars of war go beyond personal suffering. It has been noted that after the Second Word War, both the German and French nations were left with 'deep psychological scars', the former because of the Nazi atrocities and from losing the war, and the latter because of surrendering to the Germans in 1940 and the ensuing collaboration by the Vichy Regime (Marwick, 1988). But both Germany and France have survived, al-be-it that the former was divided for over 40 years but is also the economic powerhouse of Europe. Furthermore, notwithstanding the undoubtedly horrendous mental distress the Holocaust caused for all too many, some survivors did survive surprisingly psychologically undamaged or at least not so damaged as to fail to go on to lead successful lives.[4]

Whether positive or negative, the consequences of a social crisis can be immediate or delayed, short-lasting or prolonged. As I continue to write this book (mid-2023), the conflict continues in Ukraine. Russia's 2022 invasion of Ukraine, now in its second year, already hundreds of thousands of people have died, towns and cities have been destroyed, millions of Ukrainians have been displaced with many leaving their country, and up to one million residents and citizens have left Russia, vast amounts of armaments used by both sides have been used at a cost of US$ billions, and the global economy slumped not long after the war started and remains in a trough having. It is too early to calculate precisely how much harm is being done to the mental health of combatants and civilians. What is certain is that there will have been much psychological suffering and much of this suffering will not suddenly abate whenever the war ends. Furthermore, it is likely more psychological suffering will surface after that date.

There are multiple threats to maintaining psychological stability from all conflicts, especially on the scale of the war in Ukraine. War-affected civilians as well as combatants are prone to undiagnosed but not necessarily negligible amounts of psychological suffering. Some will receive a psychiatric diagnosis of, for example, anxiety, depression, or PTSD. Moreover, Russia's invasion of the internationally recognised – including previously by Russia – Ukrainian borders began in 2014, and there is evidence of deteriorating mental well-being amongst Ukrainians caught up in fighting over the ensuing years What is also recognisable from these years of war in Ukraine, as is in other conflicts, are the opposite effects to that of mental travails.

A sizeable proportion of Ukrainian's military force is made up of civilians (Russia also mobilised reservists and paramilitary mercenaries from the 'Wagner Group' and convicts). According to psychologist Richard Bryant and his colleagues (Bryant *et al.*, 2022), civilian combatants are indeed at risk of psychological deterioration, but also may experience a surge in their mental well-being. Civilians defending their country may have beneficial effects psychologically because of the sense of purpose it provides. This psychological benefit may, however, reduce in proportion to the increased risk to corporeal integrity and endurance. Furthermore, in this conflict, civilians, reservists, and convicts have been drafted without adequate training. They face the fighting without the skills developed by established militaries. This leaves them even vulnerable more vulnerable to physical and psychological damage if not death than military regulars. There is also the problem for both sides in the conflict of having recruited people unsuitable or armed action. The unsuitability may be due to age, physical prowess, or psychological solidity. Richard Bryant and his colleagues point to yet another risk factor for 'new' recruits:

> [N]ew recruits into the military might not experience the same sense of unit cohesion as longer-serving personnel, which is relevant because unit cohesion can be protective against PTSD.
>
> (Bryant *et al.*, 2022, p.346)

There are further psychological pressures placed all Ukrainian military personnel with the fracturing of social ties following the mass fleeing of relatives. As Bryant and his colleagues comment, social connectedness is a key protective buffer to the effects of stress. If friends and family have remained in the country they may face attacks from the enemy, and their worries add to those of the combatants.

Those remaining to fight are faced with severe threats without the protective effects of their social support systems. For those who have remained in Ukraine to fight, these risks might be heightened by ongoing worries about the safety and well-being of family members who have fled the country. Technology may soften some of these stressors or possibly inflame concerns. Mobile phones provide the opportunity for maintaining connectedness or reconnecting with loved ones and thereby supply reciprocal emotions between loved ones. But communication also provides the opportunity for further worry because of the knowledge of each other's troubles.

Pre-existing Mental Health Crisis

Although the COVID-pandemic worsened the situation regarding mental well-being, there were reports of a crisis of psychological suffering before the COVID-19 crisis. In a policy briefing by the United Nations in May 2020, it is stated that up to 85% of people with 'mental health conditions' who live in low-and middle-income countries do not have access to formal services and treatments (United Nations, 2020). Illustrating this deficit, the report refers to the extremely low number of mental health professionals there are to provide these services and treatments (less than one for every 10,000 people globally). What is also mentioned in the report is the level of human rights violations against people diagnosed with severe mental health disorders, declaring that it is widespread in all countries of the world. What the United Nations also declares is that after a few months of the pandemic psychological distress had also become widespread. Furthermore, there is an explicit acceptance of the interrelationship between personal (psychological) well-being and the well-being of society, and that the pandemic had already enfeebled both. The havoc caused by the pandemic on the economy and health systems made people more fearful and despondent, and as psychological solidity decreased so did the stability of society (Rahman *et al.*, 2020).

So, the pandemic seemingly worsened the existing global mental health crisis. An example of data suggesting that the COVID-19 pandemic increasing the crisis for mental health in the UK is provided by the Royal College of Psychiatry. According to the Royal College of Psychiatry using data obtained from the National Health Service for the period January 2021 and December of that year, there was a total of 4.3 million referrals to mental health services in England alone. This represented the highest number of referrals ever recorded in that country. The psychiatric conditions associated with these referrals encompassed various addictions, anxiety, depression, and eating disorders. This apparent mental health crisis then led to a crisis in providing not only facilities and treatments but initial consultations for assessment of need (Royal College of Psychiatrists, 2022).

Prescriptions for antidepressants in England had been rising for years in England before the arrival of COVID-19. In the second year of the pandemic, the number of antidepressant drugs prescribed in England is estimated to have more than 83 million. By then nearly half a million more adults were taking these drugs, an increase of over 5% on the previous year. There had also been an increase in the number of antidepressant prescriptions for children and teenagers (National Health Service Business Services Authority, 2022). The COVID-19 pandemic has therefore contributed to, but had not been the primary cause of, an apparent epidemic of misery that pharmaceuticals were considered by general practitioners and psychiatrists as either the most suitable treatment or the only practical one available.

Certainly, there has been a huge rise in the diagnosis of mental disorders in developed countries, and increasingly in emergent and undeveloped countries. Psychiatric researchers Fuller Torrey and Judy Miller (2002) argue that there is an ongoing but unacknowledged 'plague' of mental disorder, but that this began centuries ago. For Torrey and Miller medicalisation and constructionist theses that regard madness as 'made up' are misplaced. For them, mental disorder is not only real but an unappreciated and genuine 'plague'. The incidence of what they surmise is 'brain-based insanity' has increased in the last three centuries due to major changes in where and how people live. That is, the societal circumstances of humans over 300 years have altered dramatically. Specifically, there has not been a drift but a surge in populations moving from the countryside to the cities.

Urbanisation, argue Torrey and Miller, is principally responsible for the 'invisible plague' of mental disorder. Although they examined only records relating to mental disorder in England, Ireland, Canada, and the USA, the implication is that the process of urbanisation that has occurred worldwide has contributed to the mental disorder 'plague'. Torrey and Miller insist upon the biological reality of insanity. For example, schizophrenia, for them, may be connected to exposure to the 'infective agents' (causative candidates, they suggest, are disease, diet, and alcohol) that are readily formed and easily disseminated in urban environments, especially those that are densely packed with humans and animals.

But so far research over hundreds of years, into the biological basis of the hundreds of mental disorders listed in the psychiatric manuals has failed, except for a very few exceptions, to move beyond conjecture. This is yet not objective, irrefutable proof that schizophrenia is always if ever essentially based in biology.

Unadulterated biological deterministic explanations for the cause of diagnosed mental disorders, however, continue. According to a study conducted by an international team of researchers, problems with the ability of the brain to prune itself of unnecessary synaptic connections may be the origin of a wide range of mental disorders that are diagnosed in adolescence and may continue into adulthood (Xie *et al.*, 2023). Depression, anxiety, and behavioural disorders, such as attention deficit hyperactivity disorder are examples of these disorders, these researchers claim. These researchers also suggest that defective cerebral trimming may be the reason why an individual is diagnosed with multiple mental disorders. Apart from this research paying virtually no due heed to crucial cultural factors that affect the psychological development and performance of young people, the suggestion that a broad biological process in the brain can malfunction in such a specific way as to produce a 'pruned' mental disorder labels illogical. Moreover, there is an abundance of evidence that brain development, including the manner of synaptic growth, persistence, decay, and death, is affected by social and physical environments in childhood (Tooley *et al.*, 2021).

The exponential rise in self and professional diagnosis of 'mental health problems' and 'mental disorders' coincides with an avowed centuries-long 'civilising' of society (Pinker, 2011). Torrey and Miller (2002) affirm that urbanisation, condensed living conditions, and global trade, are notable upshots of advancing civilisation. They have also, they posit, played a major role in creating a plague of mental disorder. But, if society is so civilised, then logically its psychologically toxic elements would have dissolved or at least be diminished.

A fundamental feature of neoliberal capitalism is inequality. Epidemiologists Richard Wilkinson and Kate Pickett (2010; 2018) argue that there has been a conspicuous upturn in the diagnosis mental disorder coinciding with a conspicuous upturn in inequality. They are not questioning the legitimacy of mental disorder diagnoses. Following extensive and in-depth epidemiological analysis of historical trends, they conclude that, for example, there has been an exponential rise in social anxiety paralleling a widening of the gap between the material well-off and the materially impoverished.

While Wilkinson and Pickett's reasoning relies on there being a rise in authentic mental disorder, they also accept that there has been inappropriate medicalisation of psychological suffering. They also cite the example of 'social anxiety'. It is, they argue, credible to consider that deleterious social circumstances proliferate anxiousness, but reconfiguring shyness and feelings of inferiority *per se* as symptoms of mental disorder is not credible. Social anxiety for Wilkinson and Pickett is societal in origin. It is related directly to significant structural disparities. But there is also a matter of perception at the level of the individual. There is sensitivity about self-worth largely based on discernment about economic social status. This perceptual sensitivity Wilkinson and Pickett describe as 'social evaluative threat'. People persistently peruse their social surroundings and scrutinise those with whom they associate directly for signifiers to establish where they fit in a money-orientated pecking order. Material wealth is signifying a host of other elements of high status. It is indicative of personal power, privilege, and pleasure.

In societies with reduced inequality, the happiness quotient rises providing basic needs are satisfied (Wilkinson and Pickett, 2010; 2018). These needs are having enough nutrition, adequate housing, safety from violence and exploitation, sufficient social support, and opportunities to be creative. When people have these needs accommodated, and they do not experience gross differences in income and possessions, there is a strong association with increased life satisfaction compared to that of people who are relatively much better off in material terms but live in an unequal society. Furthermore, social trust and interpersonal altruism are lower in materially unbalanced societies compared to those that are more materially balanced. But of course, there are paradoxes and complexities here as well.

Political scientist Benjamin Radcliff has reviewed the evidence on trust and happiness affiliation. The evidence indicates that countries that are rated as having high trust such as Finland tend also measure highly on levels of happiness. Trust allows for the strengthening of interpersonal and community connectivity. People who believe they can trust each other and, for example. receive support when needed and that social systems are in place that reduce the risk of being a victim of crime, can spend less emotional energy on worrying about impending woes. That leaves more emotional energy for enjoyment. Trust is improved when people perceive a society not to be riddled with a disproportionate distribution of resources. There is also evidence that inequality counts when it comes to happiness. In countries where there a high degree of happiness equality, there is a raising of happiness overall in the population. Political scientist Benjamin Radcliff's conclusion on the correlation between trustfulness and happiness equality:

> So if more trust produces more happiness equality, and more happiness equality means higher levels of happiness itself, then trust should, once again, promote greater happiness.
>
> (Radcliff, 2022)

The paradox regarding trust is that capitalism relies on businesses being able to operate in a trustful environment whereby mutual obligations are assured, yet the more capitalism 'matures' (that is, the further neoliberal tenets are embedded in its practices), trust and altruism are subverted by self-serving profit-making.

The complexity regarding trust, material inequality, and life satisfaction is explained by economist and theologian Johan Graafland and economist Bjorn Lous:

> [L]ife satisfaction inequality has a significant diminishing effect on trust and should therefore be considered equally with income inequality when it comes to its impact on trust.
>
> (Graafland and Lous, 2019, p.1732)

What Graafland and Lous are pointing out is that there is not a linear connection between inequality, happiness, and trust. They argue that lower inequality and a higher level of life satisfaction, apart from fairness being morally valuable, contribute to economic growth because it enhances trust.

It would seem that not persistently and steadfastly securing trust in all or at least most of its operations, capitalism triggers yet another dysfunctional facet that undermines its own endurance. Conflicts and contagions would also seem to be major dysfunctional facets for any economic system that relies on trust and certainly not seem functional for the fairer distribution of happiness. Graafland and Lous were writing before the arrival of COVID-19. This contagion caused a global crisis in capitalism and put trust further to the test. Trustfulness wavered. Trust improved within in certain communities and in expert opinion may well have risen but not consistently. Trust in politicians faltered in at the height of the pandemic and subsequently dipped markedly. Trust in the capitalist enterprise also swerved.

Money matters for mental health. Wilkinson and Pickett give the example of the owners and managers of big business receiving salaries hundreds of times greater than the lowest-paid employees in the same company and taking large bonuses. Self-perceptions of personal worth correspond to these payments. The more you receive financially, the greater your self-worth. Those at the bottom of the payment pyramid have lower self-esteem and worse physical and psychological health. Awareness of wealth differentiation is unavoidable. In a globalised technological world, there is virtually no avoiding the realisation that some people are tremendously rich while others were horrendously poor. There is virtually no avoiding the realisation that much of a country's wealth in most countries is in the hands of a tiny minority of people. There is virtually no avoiding the realisation that much of the wealth of the world is located in Western countries. Perhaps there is less realisation that most of the wealth of the world is in the hands of an international elite.

The International Monetary Fund (IMF) is a financial agency of the United Nations. It has a declared aim of achieving sustainable growth and prosperity for all (IMF, 2023). A sizeable and possibly insurmountable obstacle to achieving that aim is inequality. Inequality is built-in to the economic system supported by the IMF. Inequality, rather than sustaining economic growth and prosperity 'for all', serves the minority at the expense of the majority. The physical, psychological, and ethical overheads from inequality are substantial. Economic growth and prosperity is a parochial ambition, a goal blind-sided by financial considerations rather than regarding humanity's achievements to be better measured against sustainable growth and prosperity in, for example, personal creativity, interpersonal connectivity, and societal sanity.

It's not as though the IMF doesn't realise there is a problem with inequality. In a report published by the International monetary fund in 2022 using data supplied by the *World Inequality Database* (Chancel *et al.*, 2021), global inequalities are stated to be in 'bad shape' (Stanley, 2022). As a consequence of economic deregulation and liberalisation, inequalities in wealth and income have risen steeply in most countries since the 1980s. The most marked divisions in wealth and income since that time have occurred in the USA, Russia, and India. By the 2020s, the richest 10% of the global population owned nearly 200 times that of the poorest 50%. More than half of all income globally goes to 10% of the population. From the data extracted from the World Inequality Database, the IMF both accepts and asserts that the already bad shape of inequalities is worsening.

It is, however, more accurate to describe equalities to be in bad shape because inequalities are in good shape in the sense that they have not only been preserved but are persevering. The reason the plural 'inequalities' is adopted in the report is because there is a reference to other disparities than that of wealth, although all of these are associated with financial security or insecurity. For example, fairness in income allocation and access to employment for women continues to be in bad shape. Another example is the unfairness in the ownership of land and business. A third example is ecological inequality with poor nations and poor communities within rich countries taking the brunt of pollutants from the dense flow of traffic and industry input because they live and work in unregulated environments. The exposure to pollution is made all the worse by the shift of most of the world's population into dense and unfettered and frequently festering urbanised areas. Some parts of the world are heading towards making personal, public, and commercial transportation largely or wholly electric thereby reducing exposure to toxins for those living and working in the vicinity (but not necessarily for those living and working where the electricity is produced). Some parts of the world are managing to make their industries much more environmentally friendly by producing fewer pollutants from the use of sustainable energy and manufacturing long-lasting or recyclable goods (unless they are disingenuously 'green washing' as opposed to genuinely 'going green'). Many parts of the world are not managing to reduce the number of diesel vehicles or unfiltered release of chemicals into the air from heavy manufacturing and waste disposal sites (much of which may be producing products for and taking the waste from richer and purportedly 'greener' parts of the world).

According to the *World Inequality Database* (Chancel *et al.*, 2021), the COVID-19 pandemic contributed to the splaying of disproportion in wealth. The data from this source were published in December of 2021. This was before the invasion of Ukraine by Russia. Therefore, the conclusions of *World Inequality Database at this stage* do not include the impact of the war on the global economy and the likely effect of further worsening the already terrible state of equality. One conclusion from the *World Inequality Database*'s report that is highly relevant to the mitigation of inequity, and by implication many other societal insanities and social crises, is the degree to which governments are proactive. During the COVID-19 pandemic, there were marked differences in how proactive governments decided to be in relation to poverty. *Lead author of the World Inequality Database 's global study of inequality* **Lucas Chancel**, *reflects on the key lesson learned:*

> The COVID crisis has exacerbated inequalities between the very wealthy and the rest of the population. Yet, in rich countries, government intervention prevented a massive rise in poverty, this was not the case in poor countries….. [I]nequality is always a political choice.
>
> (Chancel *et al.*, 2021)

Inequality is not an inevitability, it is not an inherent element of the human condition, it is not a necessary facet of a functional society. Capitalism does generate inequalities, but the immensity of current disparities is not necessary and is dysfunctional. It is also immoral to have so many people in the world scraping an existence, condemned to lingering maladies and premature expiration while others are wallowing in the world's resources for much longer and with much less risk of being distracted by sickness from enjoying their prosperousness. Global society in the 21st century is infused with such indecent concomitant absurdities of obesity and famishment, average lifespans of not much over 50 years in some locales and well over 80 years elsewhere, and millions of children having to work to keep them and their families alive and dying from preventable and curable diseases while others enjoy prolonged and protected childhoods.

So, low wages, little power, and paltry prestige, all appear to exacerbate physical and psychological morbidity and a reduction in lifespan. But levels of happiness (life satisfaction) may vacillate depending on perceptions of equality. Moreover, impoverishment (but not starvation, homelessness, or being a victim of, for example, violence), in itself may not be always linkable to unhappiness. Also, happiness is also not always linkable to psychological suffering. Psychological suffering does not necessarily lead to dysfunction. Satisfaction with life may be gained by enduring dissatisfactions. Delayed gratification is a common feature of human performance in modern society, enabling greater rewards through, for example, passing examinations, undergoing lengthy training, undertaking physically challenging feats, and rearing children.

Trust is interconnected with psychological solidity and life satisfaction. Altruism is also linked to happiness and mental well-being. Both trust and altruism overlap with the signs of societal sanity that include kindliness, cooperativeness, truthfulness, and resilience. There is also overlap between altruism, kindness, and prosocial performances. To remind, the reader, human 'performance' as it is defined in this book is not only referring to behaviours. Behaviour is the 'doing' aspect of how humans operate. But along with behaviours, emotions and cognitions contribute to the composition and comprehension of humans. Much of the literature ascribes only 'behaviour' when referring to prosocial performance. However, there is the inference that emotions and cognitions are implicated. There is also a tendency in the literature to conflate the terms altruism and prosocial behaviour. I am following psychologist Nancy Eisenberg's (1982) definition by including altruism, kindness, and cooperation as the main components of prosocial behaviours, but replacing 'behaviour' with 'performance'. This applies to the synonyms, divisions, and associated concepts of these three core conditions of human performance (this includes trust). However, consistency is not necessarily a hallmark of my use of these terms.

Acts of altruism vary widely and do the motivations that lead to prosocial behaviour (Ricard, 2018). Examples include volunteering to help in a charity shop, donating blood or giving donations to fund emergency services when disasters occur such as hurricanes, earthquakes strike, and famines. But, low-key altruistic acts, similar to those that display kindness and cooperation, occur regularly and are often hardly noticed by either the donor or receiver.

Some of these acts may be motivated by an unpretentious and self-less conscious desire or unconscious impulse to help. Some of these acts may be motivated by self-interest whereby direct reciprocation is expected or by indirect self-interest whereby there is the implication that one of the communities in which the donor belongs will benefit in the future. From an evolutionary perspective whatever the act and whatever the supposed motivation, altruism is enhancing the chances of survival and reproduction of both the donor and receiver, therefore it is in everyone's interest to engage in prosocial behaviour. In altruistic exchanges, there is also a 'cost-benefit' assessment, and that also may be conscious or unconscious. However, this assessment is complex. It may involve, for example, considering how close in genetic terms the donor regards him/herself is to the receiver, whether there will be any benefit directly or indirectly, and whether the act will be accepted or rejected.

The study of altruism in relation to inequality and therefore in relation to mental health, has provided curious results. For example, there is much empirical evidence to indicate that the rich are less generous than the poor. There are many studies that suggest there is an enlarging of this difference in highly economically unequal countries. However, the results from research conducted by sociologists Yen-Sheng Chiang and Jacqueline Chen (2019) imply that where the level of inequality is elevated this tends to mitigate the difference.

The opposite of altruism is not selfishness but performances that protect and promote the ego (altruistic acts can do this) and are damaging to other people and/or society. It may be that acts appear altruistic the benefit from them is designed only to support the egotistical gain of the 'donor' at the expense of the 'receiver' which may be society. Extreme anti-altruism is narcissism. There are, however, two types of narcissism. There is personal narcissistic performance and cultural narcissism. While individuals can be motivated to act narcissistically, narcissistic cultures will craft and fuel wholesale narcissism. Wilkinson and Pickett (2018) regard personal narcissism as an ego-defence mechanism in those with low self-worth resulting from daily experiences of belittlement, shaming, rejection, deprivation, and powerlessness. Low self-worth is much more likely among people at the bottom of the social hierarchy. The reaction of some people in this category may be to overindulge the self and manufacture or exaggerate the value of achievements. But Wilkinson and Picket, point out that narcissism is operative and apparent in those at the top end of the social hierarchy. Excessive egocentricity, cupidity, conceit, and manipulativeness, may have enabled the rich and powerful to become privileged and powerful, and once in that position allow them to administer belittlement, shaming, and rejection to uphold and inflate their standing. According to Wilkinson and Pickett, 'status anxiety' is common in cultures with inequality as a staple feature.

What Wilkinson and Pickett (2018) also acknowledge are the background stimuli for anti-altruism and narcissism. A culture that generates and congratulates individualism, avarice, commodification, and consumerism, will also foment and reward complementary individual and organisational performances. Successful individuals in this setting may display the symptoms of narcissism and its associated personality disorder of psychopathy. A successful business may also exhibit these characteristics. Successful narcissistic and psychopathic people and narcissistic businesses may be co-dependent. That is, such businesses be found to have employed and promoted staff who if assessed clinically would reveal narcissistic or psychopathic traits in a greater number than their would-be competitors (Babiak and Hare, 2019).

Wilkinson and Picket (2018), however, make it clear that they do not subscribe to the notion that there is an epidemic of narcissism and psychopathy. Most people are not narcissists or psychopaths. But they do subscribe to the notion that there are epidemics of real mental disorders, notably depression and anxiety, and that this has societal roots. They do acknowledge the role of biology but that cause and effect are reversed. That is, scans that show alterations in neurological structures and processes are demonstrating the effects of detrimental societal factors, a predominant one for Wilkinson and Picket being in a low position with a highly divergent, rigid, and unfair, social hierarchy.

In a prescient publication, the historian and social critic Christopher Lasch suggested that the culture of USA from the 19th century onwards has been inherently narcissistic. His book titled 'The Culture of Narcissism', was published in 1979. Since then, the culture of narcissism has arguably spread globally through the global spread of a common economic system. For Lasch this is not normal. Humans have lived in groups for most of their history as a species that have not been based on selfishness, self-importance, self-promotion, and celebrity.

Summary

In the previous chapter, the social crises of contagions and conflicts (were discussed). In this chapter, the consequences for mental health of these catastrophic events have been explored. These consequences are more far-reaching than how they affect mental well-being. They have major effects on the functioning and formation of society. But it is also the case that how society is formed and how it functions impacts mental health and furnishes contagions and conflicts.

Homo Erectus was a hominin, a creature who evolved away from other gatherer and scavenger hominin lineages to become a savannah predator and emigrate from Africa. This species began about two million years ago and died out over 100,000 years ago (Gee, 2021). Homo erectus was sociable, a maker of fire, a cook, and a designer of a primitive 'hand axe' tool. So far, what this tool was used for has not been discerned. But why should such an artefact have a purpose? Although it is the correct shape to fit in a hand, why has it been referred to as an 'axe' when there is no evidence that it has been used for chopping or slicing. Finding functionality may be more of a function of faulty thinking about evolutionary outcomes and an intellectual artefact of modern humans. It could be that some things do not have or need a purpose. There is a parallel to be drawn with the search for 'faults' to explain and construct mental disorders. Maybe there isn't a 'fault' to be found. Maybe there isn't a mental health crisis to be found. This latter point is explored in the next chapter.

Notes

1 Chapter 4 examines further the issue of personal and social resilience.
2 The 'height' of the COVID-19 pandemic here is referring to the various heightened levels of infection that were recorded over the two-year period from early 2020 to late 2021. However, at the time of writing (mid-2023) both original and novel variants of the SARS-CoV-2 continue to infect millions of people globally. At the beginning of 2023, a new wave of COVID-19 was reported to be spreading rapidly in China (Kleczkowski, 2023).
3 With the intention of reminding the reader (and the author) but at the risk of irritating the reader, the core themes of the book surface regularly throughout the book. The one mentioned here is that of 'paradox'. That is, all forms of existence (humans, animals, nature, the universe, and all of its atomical makeup) are replete with contradictions. Human inspired sense and nonsense coexist, general relativity theory and quantum standard model are (as yet) incompatible but nevertheless cohabit in contemporary physics.
4 More on how survivors coped after the Holocaust in discussed in Chapter 4.

References

Albrecht G, Sartore G, Connor L, Higginbotham N, Freeman S, Kelly B, Stain H, Tonna A and Pollard G (2007) The Distress Caused by Environmental Change. *Australian Psychiatry*, 15(Supplement 1), pp.S95–S98.

Amnesty International (2004) *Clouds of Injustice: Bhopal Disaster 20 Years On*. London: Amnesty International.

Babiak P and Hare R (2019) (revised edition) *Snakes in Suits, Revised Edition: Understanding and Surviving the Psychopaths in Your Office*. New York: Harper Business.

Bell P (2015) Why Is Loneliness Becoming a Major Issue Among Men Who Aren't Elderly? Huffington Post, 7th October. https://www.huffingtonpost.co.uk/2014/11/05/loneliness-in-men-talking-about-it_n_6105402.html [accessed 12th May, 2023]

British Association for Counselling and Psychotherapy (2020) Mental Health Impact of Climate Change. London: BACP. https://www.bacp.co.uk/news/news-from-bacp/2020/15-october-mental-health-impact-of-climate-change/ [accessed 3rd January, 2022]

Bryant R, Schnurr P and Pedlar D (2022) Addressing the Mental Health Needs of Civilian Combatants in Ukraine. *The Lancet Psychiatry*, 9(5), pp.346–347.

Bulletin of the Atomic Scientists (2023) A Time of Unprecedented Danger: It Is 90 Seconds to Midnight. The Bulletin Science and Security Board. https://thebulletin.org/doomsday-clock/current-time/ [accessed 25th January, 2023]

Butterworth B (2021) Police Officers Facing Mental Health Crisis [Main Article Has the Headline 'Officers under Pressure 'Like Never Before' Due to Workload']. The i, [British newspaper] 26th July, 2021.

Centers for Disease Control and Prevention (2013) About Severe Acute Respiratory Syndrome (SARS). https://www.cdc.gov/sars/about/index.html [accessed 20th January, 2023].

Chancel L, Piketty T, Saez E and Zucman K (2021) World Inequality Report 2022. World Inequality Database. https://wir2022.wid.world/ [accessed 9th March, 2023]

Chiang Y and Chen J (2019) Does Inequality Cause a Difference in Altruism Between the Rich and the Poor? Evidence from a Laboratory Experiment. *Social Indicators Research*, 144(1), pp.73–95.

Cianconi P, Betrò S and Janiri L (2020) The Impact of Climate Change on Mental Health: A Systematic Descriptive Review. *Frontiers in Psychiatry*, 11(74), 6th March. https://www.frontiersin.org/articles/10.3389/fpsyt.2020.00074/full [accessed 10th August, 2021]

Clayton S (2021) Climate Change and Mental Health. *Current Environmental Health Reports*, 8(1), pp.1–6.

Committee on the Medical Effects of Air Pollutants (2022) *Cognitive Decline, Dementia and Air Pollution. Committee on the Medical Effects of Air Pollutants.* London: UK Health Security Agency.

Das-Munshi J, Changa C, Bakolis I, Broadbent M, Dregan A, Hotopf M, Morgan C and Stewart R (2021) All-Cause and Cause-Specific Mortality in People with Mental Disorders and Intellectual Disabilities, Before and During the COVID-19 Pandemic: Cohort Study. The Lancet Regional Health – Europe, 7th October, 100228. https://www.thelancet.com/journals/lanepe/article/PIIS2666-7762(21)00214-3/fulltext [accessed 10th October, 2021].

Davis S (2020) 'Sheer Fear': Mental Health Impacts of Covid-19 Come to Fore. *The Guardian*, 15th August, 2020.

D'Silva T (2006) *The Black Box of Bhopal: A Closer Look at the World's Deadliest Industrial Accident.* Bloomington, IN: Trafford.

Duhon H (2014 Bhopal: A Root Cause Analysis of the Deadliest Industrial Accident in History. *Journal of Petroleum Technology*, 2nd May. https://jpt.spe.org/bhopal-root-cause-analysis-deadliest-industrial-accident-history [accessed 10th January, 2023]

Eisenberg N (1982) (editor) *The Development of Prosocial Behavior.* New York: Academic Press.

Fancourt D, Steptoe A and Bradbury A (2022) *Tracking the Psychological and Social Consequences of the COVID-19 Pandemic across the UK Population: Findings, Impact, and Recommendations from the COVID-19 Social Study (March 2020 – April 2022).* London: University College London.

Figueroa R, Cortés P, Marín H, Vergés A, Gillibrand R and Repetto P (2022) The ABCDE Psychological First Aid Intervention Decreases Early PTSD Symptoms But Does Not Prevent It: Results of a Randomized-Controlled Trial. *European Journal of Psychotraumatology*, 13(1), 2031829. https://www.ncbi.nlm.nih.gov/pmc/articles/PMC8890535/ [accessed 9th January, 2023]

Forstmeier A, Hal E, Auerbach M, Maercker A and Brom D (2020) Life Review Therapy for Holocaust Survivors (LRT-HS): Study Protocol for a Randomised Controlled Trial. *BioMed Central Psychiatry*, 20, p.186. https://bmcpsychiatry.biomedcentral.com/articles/10.1186/s12888-020-02600-5 [accessed 30th January, 2023]

Gee H (2021) *A (Very) Short History of Life on Earth*. London: Picador.

Goldman E and Galea S (2014) Mental Health Consequences of Disasters. *Annual Review of Public Health*, 35, pp.169–183.

Graafland J and Lous B (2019) Income Inequality, Life Satisfaction Inequality and Trust: A Cross Country Panel Analysis. *Journal of Happiness Studies*, 20(6), pp.1717–1737.

Gray R (2019) Covered up by a Secretive Soviet Union at the Time, the True Number of Deaths and Illnesses Caused by the Nuclear Accident are Only Now Becoming Clear. BBC Future, 26th July. https://www.bbc.com/future/article/20190725-will-we-ever-know-chernobyls-true-death-toll [accessed 27th January, 2023]

Greenberg N, Weston D, Hall C, Caulfield T, Williamson V and Fong K (2021) Mental Health of Staff Working in Intensive Care During Covid-19. *Occupational Medicine*, 71(2), pp.62–67.

Greene T, Harju-Seppänen J, Adeniji M, Steel C, Grey N, Brewin C, Bloomfield M and Billings J (2021) Predictors and Rates of PTSD, Depression and Anxiety in UK Frontline Health and Social Care Workers During COVID-19. *European Journal of Psychotraumatology*, 12(1). https://www.tandfonline.com/doi/full/10.1080/20008198.2021.1882781 [accessed 1st October, 2021]

Greenpeace (2006) (revised edition) *The Chernobyl Catastrophe: Consequences on Human Health*. Amsterdam: Greenpeace.

Hass A (1995) *The Aftermath: Living with the Holocaust*. New York: Cambridge University Press, 1995.

Hickman C, Marks E, Pihkala P, Clayton C, Lewandowski E, Mayall E, Wray B, Mellor C and Susteren L (2021) Climate Anxiety in Children and Young People and their Beliefs about Government Responses to Climate Change: A Global Survey. *The Lancet Planetary Health*, 5(12), pp.e863–e873.

Holmes E, O'Connor R, Perry V, Tracey I, Wessely S, Arseneault L, Ballard C, Christensen H, Silver R, Everall I, Ford T, John A, Kabir T, King K, Madan I, Michie S, Przybylski A, Shafran R, Sweeney A, Worthman C, Yardley L, Cowan K, Cope C, Hotopf M, Bullmore E (2020) Multidisciplinary Research Priorities for the COVID-19 Pandemic: A Call for Action for Mental Health Science. *The Lancet*, 7(6), pp.547–560.

Hudson K (2013) Hiroshima – the Truth About the Bombing. Campaign for Nuclear Disarmament. https://cnduk.org/hiroshima-the-truth-about-the-bombing/ [accessed 10th February, 2023]

International Atomic Energy Agency (2023) Frequently Asked Chernobyl Questions. https://www.iaea.org/newscenter/focus/chernobyl/faqs [accessed 27th January, 2023]

International Monetary Fund (2023) IMF-at-a-Glance. https://www.imf.org/en/About/Factsheets/IMF-at-a-Glance [accessed 10th March, 2023]

International Panel on Climate Change (2022) Climate Change 2022: Impacts, Adaptation and Vulnerability. Working Group II Contribution to the IPCC Sixth Assessment Report. Geneva: International Panel on Climate Change.

Ipsos MORI (2021) State of the Nation: Understanding Public Attitudes to the Early Years. London: Royal Foundation of The Duke and Duchess of Cambridge. https://royalfoundation.com/understanding-public-attitudes-to-the-early-years/ [accessed 25th October, 2021]Johnson D and Kendall C (2020) Student Mental Health: 'I Am Living in a Bubble of One'. BBC News, 9th December. https://www.bbc.co.uk/news/education-55105044 [accessed 19th October, 2021]

King's College London News (2021) Exposure to Air Pollution Linked with Increased Mental Health Service-Use, New Study Finds. https://www.kcl.ac.uk/news/exposure-to-air-pollution-linked-with-increased-mental-health-service-use-new-study-finds [accessed 20th February, 2023]

Kleczkowski A (2023) COVID is Running Rampant in China – But Herd Immunity Remains Elusive. The Conversation, 23rd January. https://theconversation.com/covid-is-running-rampant-in-china-but-herd-immunity-remains-elusive-197454 [accessed 24th January, 2023].

Kobayashi T, Maeda M, Nakayama C, Takebayashi Y, Sato H, Setou N, Momoi M, Horikoshi N, Yasumura A and O Hitoshi (2022) Disaster Resilience Reduces Radiation-Related Anxiety Among Affected People 10 Years After the Fukushima Daiichi Nuclear Power Plant Accident. *Frontiers Public Health*, 14th July, 10(839442). file:///C:/Users/campb/Downloads/fpubh-10–839442.pdf [accessed 29th January, 2023]

LaCapra D (2001) *Writing History, Writing Trauma*. Baltimore, MD: Johns Hopkins University Press.

Lasch C (1979) *The Culture of Narcissism: American Life in an Age of Diminishing Expectations*. New York: Norton.

Lee A, Wong J, McAlonan G, Cheung V, Cheung C, Sham P, Chu CM Wong P, Tsang K and Chua S (2007) Stress and Psychological Distress Among SARS Survivors 1 Year After the Outbreak. *Canadian Journal of Psychiatry*, 52(4), pp.233–240.

Longmuir C and Agyapon VIO (2022) Social and Mental Health Impact of Nuclear Disaster in Survivors: A Narrative Review. *Behavioral Sciences*, 11(8), p.113. https://www.ncbi.nlm.nih.gov/pmc/articles/PMC8389263/ [accessed 26th January, 2023]

Mak I, Chu C, Pan P, Yiu M, and Chan V (2009) Long-Term Psychiatric Morbidities Among SARS Survivors. *General Hospital Psychiatry*, 31(4), pp.318–326.

Makwana N (2019) Disaster and its Impact on Mental Health: A Narrative Review. *Journal of Family Medicine and Primary Care*, 8(10), pp.3090–3095.

Marmot M, Allen J, Goldblatt P, Herd E and Morrison J (2020) *Build Back Fairer: The COVID-19 Marmot Review: The Pandemic, Socioeconomic and Health Inequalities in England*. London: Institute of Health Equity.

Marshall M (2020) How COVID-19 can Damage the Brain. *Nature* 585(7825), pp.342–343.

Marwick A (1988) (editor) *Total War and Social Change*. Houndmills: Macmillan.

Masterpasqua F and Perna P (1997) (editors). *The Psychological Meaning of Chaos: Translating Theory into Practice*. Washington, DC: American Psychological Association.

Maunder R (2009) Was SARS a Mental Health Catastrophe? *General Hospital Psychiatry*, 31(4), pp.316–317.

Mazza M, DeLorenzo R, Conte C, Poletti S, Benedetta V, Bollettini I, Melloni E, Furlan R, Ciceri F, Rovere-Querini P and COVID-19 BioB Outpatient Clinic Study Group –

Benedetti F (2020) Anxiety and Depression in COVID-19 Survivors: Role of Inflammatory and Clinical Predictors. *Brain Behavior and Immunity*, 89[October], pp.594–600.

McMichael C, Barnett J and McMichael A (2012) An Ill Wind? Climate Change, Migration, and Health. *Environmental Health Perspectives*, 120(5), pp.646–654.

Morrall P (2017) *Madness: Ideas about Insanity*. Abingdon, UK: Routledge.

Mundasad S (2020) Parents Warned of 'Sharp Rise' in Eating Disorders. BBC News, 29th December. https://www.bbc.co.uk/news/health-55468632 [accessed 29th December, 2020]

Murphy R (2014) Mental Health of Survivors of 1984 Bhopal Disaster: A Continuing Challenge. *Industrial Psychiatry Journal*, 23(2), pp.86–93.

National Health Service Business Services Authority (2022) Medicines Used in Mental Health – England – 2015/16 to 2021/22. NHS Business Services Authority Statistics and Data Science, 7th July. https://www.nhsbsa.nhs.uk/statistical-collections/medicines-used-mental-health-england/medicines-used-mental-health-england-201516-202122 [accessed 10th July, 2022]

Newbury J, Stewart R, Fisher H, Beevers S, Dajnak D, Broadbent M, Pritchard M, Shiode N, Heslin M, Hammoud R, Hotopf M, Hatch S, Mudway I and Bakolis I (2021) Association Between Air Pollution Exposure and Mental Health Service Use Among Individuals with First Presentations of Psychotic and Mood Disorders: Retrospective Cohort Study. *The British Journal of Psychiatry*, 219(6), pp.678–685.

NHS Digital (2020) *Survey Conducted in July 2020 Shows One in Six Children Having a Probable Mental Disorder*. Leeds: The Health and Social Care Information Centre.

Ohta Y, Mine M, Wakasugi M, Yoshimine E, Himuro Y, Yoneda M, Yamaguchi S, Mikita A and Morikawa T (2000) Psychological Effect of the Nagasaki Atomic Bombing on Survivors After Half a Century. *Psychiatry and Clinical Neurosciences*, 54(1), pp.97–103.

Patterson R *et al.* [56 authors] (2020) The Emerging Spectrum of COVID-19 Neurology: Clinical, Radiological and Laboratory Findings. Brain, 8th July. https://academic.oup.com/brain/advance-article/doi/10.1093/brain/awaa240/5868408 [accessed 15th August, 2020]

Pinker S (2011) *The Better Angels of Our Nature: A History of Violence and Humanity*. London: Allen Lane.

Popescu S (2022) Historical Perspective: Lessons from SARS-CoV-1. *Contagion*, 7(5). https://www.contagionlive.com/view/historical-perspective-lessons-from-sars-cov-1 [accessed 20th January, 2023].

Public Health England (2020) COVID-19 Mental Health Campaign Launches. Public Health England. Press Release. https://www.gov.uk/government/news/covid-19-mental-health-campaign-launches [accessed 17th April, 2020]

Radcliff B (2022) Trusting Societies are Overall Happier – A Happiness Expert Explains Why. The Conversation, 11th May. https://theconversation.com/trusting-societies-are-overall-happier-a-happiness-expert-explains-why-177803 [accessed 8th March, 2023]

Rahman A, Naslund J, Betancourt T, Black C, Bhan A, Byansi W, Chen H, Gaynes B, Restrepo C, Gouveia L, Hamdani S, Marsch L, Petersen I, Bahar O, Shields-Zeeman L, Ssewamala F and Wainberg M (2020) The NIMH Global Mental Health Research Community and COVID-19. *The Lancet*, 7(10), pp.384–386.

Ricard M (2018) *Altruism: The Science and Psychology of Kindness*. London: Atlantic.

Rogers J, Chesney, E, Oliver D, Pollak T, McGuire P, Fusar-Poli P, Zandi M, Lewis G and David A (2020) Psychiatric and Neuropsychiatric Presentations Associated with Severe Coronavirus Infections: A Systematic Review and Meta-Analysis with Comparison to the COVID-19 Pandemic. *The Lancet*, 18th May. https://www.thelancet.com/journals/lanpsy/article/PIIS2215-0366(20)30203-0/fulltext [accessed, 12th June, 2020]

Royal College of Psychiatrists (2022) Record 4.3 Million Referrals to Specialist Mental Health Services in 2021 [Press release 15th March, 2022]. https://www.rcpsych.ac.uk/news-and-features/latest-news/detail/2022/03/15/record-4.3-million-referrals-to-specialist-mental-health-services-in-2021 [accessed 15th March, 2022]

Stanley A (2022) Global Inequalities. International Monetary Fund https://www.imf.org/en/Publications/fandd/issues/2022/03/Global-inequalities-Stanley [accessed 9th March, 2023]

Stern J (2020) This Is Not a Normal Mental-Health Disaster. The Atlantic, 7th July. https://www.theatlantic.com/health/archive/2020/07/coronavirus-special-mental-health-disaster/613510/ [accessed 27th September, 2020]

Taquet M, Geddes J, Husain M, Luciano S and Harrison P (2021) 6-Month Neurological and Psychiatric Outcomes in 236379 Survivors Of COVID-19: a Retrospective Cohort Study Using Electronic Health Records. 6th April, *Lancet Psychiatry*. https://www.thelancet.com/journals/lanpsy/article/PIIS2215-0366(21)00084-5/fulltext [accessed 7th April, 2021]

Tooley U, Bassett D and Mackey A (2021) Environmental Influences on the Pace of Brain Development. *Nature Reviews Neuroscience*, 22(6), pp.372–384.

Torrey F and Miller J (2002) *The Invisible Plague: The Rise of Mental Illness from 1750 to the Present*. New Brunswick, NJ: Rutgers University Press.

United Nations (2020) *COVID-19 and the Need for Action on Mental Health: Policy Brief*. New York: United Nations.

Weissbourd R, Batanova M, Lovison V and Torres E (2021) *Loneliness in America: How the Pandemic Has Deepened an Epidemic of Loneliness and What We Can Do About It*. Cambridge, MA: Harvard University, Graduate School of Education.

Wilkinson R and Pickett K (2010) *The Spirit Level: Why Equality is Better for Everyone*. London: Penguin.

Wilkinson R and Pickett K (2018) *The Inner Level: How More Equal Societies Reduce Stress, Restore Sanity and Improve Everyone's Wellbeing*. London: Allen Lane.

World Health Organisation (2015) Partners: Global Outbreak Alert and Response Network (GOARN). http://www.who.int/csr/disease/ebola/partners/en/ [accessed 21st January, 2023]

World Health Organisation (2017) Health Emergency and Disaster Risk Management: Mental Health and Pyschosocial Support. World Health Organization, Public Health England and Partners. https://www.who.int/hac/techguidance/preparedness/risk-management-mental-health-december2017.pdf [accessed 28th September, 2020]

World Health Organisation (2022a) COVID-19 Pandemic Triggers 25% Increase in Prevalence of Anxiety and Depression Worldwide [News Release, 22nd March] Geneva: World Health Organisation. https://www.who.int/news/item/02-03-2022-covid-19-pandemic-triggers-25-increase-in-prevalence-of-anxiety-and-depression-worldwide [accessed 7th August, 2022]

World Health Organisation (2022b) Dementia: Key Facts. https://www.who.int/news-room/fact-sheets/detail/dementia

World Health Organisation (2023) Severe Acute Respiratory Syndrome (SARS). https://www.who.int/health-topics/severe-acute-respiratory-syndrome#tab=tab_1 [accessed 19th January, 2023]

Xie C *et al.* (37 other authors) (2023) A Shared Neural Basis Underlying Psychiatric Comorbidity. *Nature Medicine*, 24th April. https://www.nature.com/articles/s41591-023-02317-4#citeas# [accessed 25th April, 2023]

Xie Y, Xu E and Al-Aly Z (2022) Risks of Mental Health Outcomes in People with Covid-19: Cohort Study. *British Medical Journal*, 376(e068993) https://www.bmj.com/content/376/bmj-2021-068993 [accessed 10th November, 2022]

Yamada M and Izumi (2002) Psychiatric Sequelae in Atomic Bomb Survivors in Hiroshima and Nagasaki Two Decades After the Explosions. *Social Psychiatry and Psychiatric Epidemiology*, 37(9), pp.409–415.

3   Mental-Healthism

Is there a mental health crisis or is there an indiscriminative, perverse, and specious obsession with mental health that can be characterised as 'mental-healthism'? The idea of 'mental-healthism'[1] combines the understanding of sincere psychological suffering with the suggestion that there is amplification if not fabrication of the negative impact on mental health from ordinary living and from extraordinary events such as social crises.

In the last chapter, evidence that widespread and lethal diseases, and periods of widespread and lethal violence, exacerbate psychological suffering was reviewed. But there is also the possibility that this evidence is misleading. Could it be that contagions and conflicts are not triggering widespread psychological suffering (including making worse existing mental distress), but that the rise is at least in part due to the undue exacerbation of the medicalisation of everyday problems and overdone media, public, academic, and political, focus on 'mental health problems'?

An example of an everyday tribulation, common when living in a city such as York, construed as a 'mental health problem' comes from the local newspaper:

> BAD busking has been affecting the mental health of staff at York's Mansion House - the home of the city's Lord Mayors… Isaac Broadbent, from the Mansion House, told a council meeting…. "Over this last year I have seen repeated exposure to the same few buskers negatively affect my employees' mental health. [uppercase in original]
>
> (Laversuch, 2020)

The common vicissitudes of life reconfigured as problems for mental health when they are revealed in the public domain via the media (but I am not suggesting bad busking in York is all that common).

This chapter starts with elaborating on the idea of mental-healthism using the exemplar of an uncommon vicissitude (the COVID-19 pandemic). Next, there is a discussion on the conceptual forerunners of mental-healthism, that is medicalisation and healthism. This is followed by a critique of the meanings associated with mental health. The contestations about the significance

DOI: 10.4324/9781003223757-4

of psychological suffering and the meaning of mental disorder are relevant to this book on social crises and mental health. This is because they reveal how personal attributes and societal circumstances collate and circumscribe how these states are experienced and acknowledged.

COVID-19 and Mental-Healthism

Many countries imposed strict lockdown measures as the seriousness of the COVID-19 pandemic began to be understood, and infection rates increased hugely followed by a huge increase in morbidity and mortality rates. Workplaces and businesses closed, and populations were legally obliged to stay at home. In many of those countries, including the UK, schools (as well as universities) also closed. This was to protect children who may already have debilitating medical conditions, and therefore vulnerable to further debilitation or death from COVID-19. It was also to protect the adult population, especially elderly relatives. A study in the USA found that children could be both symptomatic and asymptomatic carriers of the virus and therefore a potential reservoir for the transmission of present variants and the evolution of further variants (Yonker *et al.*, 2021). Exceptions were made in the UK for children of essential workers and others who were classified as socially or psychologically 'vulnerable'. Examples of these types of vulnerability included those with emotional, behavioural, and intellectual difficulties, or who were 'at risk' because of their family situations and were under the auspices of social services. Some schools remained partially open to accept children in those categories.

But there is evidence of the contrariness of the public health measures taken to try to reduce the morbidity and mortality from COVID-19. A study examining the psychological well-being of 17,000 UK school students during a COVID-19 lockdown found that one in three felt happier despite the restrictions on their movements and social contacts (Soneson *et al.*, 2022). The researchers conducting this study suggest that contributing factors to the school students' better mood include avoiding bullying, having more time to sleep and exercise, and feeling less lonely presumably because they were ensconced at home with loved ones in a non-fractions situation. A third of the students feeling happier still leaves the majority either feeling less happy or not affected by lockdown. But the researchers make the valuable observation that even though it was a minority whose mood improved, this was a surprising finding because most previous research (and much that followed) emphasised the harmful effects. They are pointing out that due attention has not been noted, or if noted not highlighted, about how even young people adapt rather than collapse in difficult circumstances. Difficult circumstances certainly are associated with the COVID-19 pandemic.

Epidemiologist Brenda Penninx and colleagues argue for caution regarding any claim of a pandemic in mental disorder. After reviewing the evidence suggesting there has been an explosion of psychological suffering, they acknowledge that COVID-19 has threatened global mental health due directly to its neuropsychiatric sequelae as well as indirectly because of the disruption the disease caused to the organisation of society. There is evidence of higher rates of symptoms of cognitive impairment, anxiety, and depression. But the threat to global mental health has not, according to Penninx and her colleagues, materialised into diagnosable mental disorder. Neither is evidence of a rise in the number of suicide or self-harm globally.

> Despite a small increase in self-reported mental health problems, this has (so far) not translated into objectively measurable increased rates of mental disorders, self-harm or suicide rates at the population level.
>
> (Penninx *et al.*, 2027, 2022)

These researchers suggest that the reason why there has not been a massive rise in diagnosable mental disorder (although non-medicalised psychological suffering has soared) is 'resilience' and 'adaptation' in the general population aided at times by governmental and community systems of support.

In a scientific briefing by the World Health Organisation, there is recognition that COVID-19 pandemic has caused much psychological suffering but also an acceptance that many 'adapted':

> The COVID-19 pandemic has had a severe impact on the mental health and wellbeing of people around the world. **While many individuals have adapted,** others have experienced mental health problems... [emphasis added].
>
> (World Health Organisation, 2022a, p.1)

Rather than the global rise in the diagnosis of mental disorders is a genuine centuries-old 'plague' as argued by Torrey and Miller (2002), it could be the product of Western-originated psychiatric, psychopharmacological, and psychotherapeutic imperialism. Psychiatric, pharmacological, and psychotherapeutic imperialism contribute to reclassifying more and more 'problems with living' as medical problems (Conrad and Slodden, 2013; Szasz, 1961; 2007). A contrasting viewpoint is that it is the genuine if disastrous outcome of a globalised 'insane' lifestyle. If the latter, then it calls into question what can be defined as madness and normality (Morrall, 2017).

Psychiatrist Ronald Pies (2020) questions whether there is a crisis in mental health or a 'pandemic' of mental disorder. He does not eschew the seriousness of symptoms signifying psychological suffering.

It is Pies's contention, however, that rarely does the genuine angst and misery associated with the fear of contracting COVID-19 or actually catching the disease, or from its social and economic detriments, warrant the diagnosis of a mental disorder using the American Psychiatric Association's Diagnostic and Statistical Manual version five criteria.

All disasters create specific vicissitudes ranging from minor distresses to sheer survival, but which inevitably become everyday problems as did COVID-19 for billions of people. Pies states he is very much aware that millions of people are suffering psychologically because of the COVID-19 pandemic. He accepts that the prevalence of symptoms of anxiety and depression had become substantially higher and that the symptoms of those with pre-existing diagnosed mental disorders such as schizophrenia ad bipolar disorder worsened. Moreover, as a psychiatrist, he deals with psychological suffering every working day, some of which he will be instrumental in diagnosing as mental disorder. There is also evidence, accepts Pies, that the pandemic may lead to serious and enduring neurological complications that are serious and enduring.

People who are seriously affected psychologically by the pandemic should, avows Pies, receive care and treatment as a priority, and long-term effects should be monitored particularly if these involve children and adolescents. This care and treatment should also be afforded to the physical and emotional toll the COVID-19 pandemic is taking on our physicians, nurses, and other front-line healthcare workers who were undergoing a physical and emotional ordeal managing the physical and psychological care and treatment of those patients infected with COVID-19.

For Pies, there are epidemiological and clinical reasons why the term 'mental health pandemic' should not be ascribed to the increase in psychological suffering associated with COVID-19. Pies also points out that the expression used in many news accounts that there is a 'mental health pandemic' is oxymoronic:

> Ironically, the term "mental health pandemic," understood in epidemiological terms, would mean something like "a worldwide outbreak of mental health!"
>
> (Pies, 2020)

What Pies states he is getting at by criticising this term is not merely indulging in semantic quibbling but how the casual misuse of language is indicative of misunderstanding in the media about what is meant by both mental health and mental ill-health. This misuse of language isn't benign, suggests Pies, but leads to misunderstanding by the public. He is also critical of how there is popular press and public conflation of 'symptoms' and 'disorder'. Again, he stresses that he is not only indicating idiomatic inaccuracy but illustrating the importance of diagnostic precision:

> A formal, clinical diagnosis of a "mental disorder" has wholly different implications—medical, legal, and psychological—than those associated with, say, a normal or adaptive response to the stress and strain of the COVID-19 pandemic.
>
> (Pies, 2020)

What Pies is pointing to Pies is the popular usage of the expression 'depression' compared to using the psychiatric appellation of 'depression' may have life-changing consequences. Labelling miserableness as a clinical condition can attract stigma, difficulties in gaining or maintaining employment, increase the cost of personal health/travel insurance, and place barriers on obtaining visas for entering foreign countries to work or as a tourist.

For Pies there is also a terminological muddle between the common use of 'anxiety' or 'stress' as opposed to how they are used in the clinical diagnosis of, for example, general anxiety disorder and post-traumatic stress disorder (PTSD). There is also a lack of distinction made in everyday conversation between 'stress' (the negative stimuli) and 'anxiety' (the negative consequence). For example, facing an examination, divorce, or disaster are 'stressors' that can cause raised heart rate and blood pressure, sweating, and flight, fight, or freeze impulses that are some of the indications of anxiety. The overall point here is that language makes a difference in the experience and perception of personal and societal phenomena.

Psychiatrist Louis Appleby is well-qualified to comment on mental health generally, suicide and homicide, in particular. Amongst other high-ranking posts connected to policies and practices concerning mental health, he is the Director of the National (UK) Confidential Inquiry into Suicide and Homicide by People with Mental Illness, and former 'Tsar' for mental health (National Director for Mental Health) and National Clinical Director for Health and Criminal Justice. He was also a key protagonist for the setting-up in 2008 an NHS initiative in England aimed at improving access to psychological therapies (IAPT) in England. The IAPT programme is intended to provide evidence-based psychological therapies to people with anxiety disorders and depression (National Institute for Health and Care Excellence, 2020).

The results from a study led by Appleby, published in 2021 indicated that despite the COVID-19 pandemic widely reported by the press, public, and professionals to have led to much psychological suffering, especially when populations were directed by the governments to isolate, suicide rates and rates of self-harm and not gone up in England in the months after the first national lockdown began in 2020 (Appleby *et al.*, 2021). In this study, mention is made of the accruing evidence that COVID-19 has harmful psychological, neurological mechanisms, and social effects, and an increase in the use of mental health helplines. Prior to the COVID-19 pandemic, there were over 6,000 deaths by suicide in the UK, and approximately 800,000 globally annually, and Appleby and his colleagues remark that the pandemic had indeed raised the risk of more suicides. These risks included the loss of social support and financial security, disruption to mental health care, emotionally and physically traumatic experiences including being seriously physically unwell, bereavement, an increase in domestic violence, and alcohol misuse. Moreover, the results from the study, according to Appleby and his colleagues, accorded with those from other high-income countries at that time (for example, from Australia, Canada, New Zealand, Norway, Peru,

Sweden, and the USA). However, what was noted in the study is the need to monitor suicide rates in the long term, and rates differ between different social groups and geographical areas within countries. For example, evidence from the USA indicated that suicide rates had increased in black but not white populations and amongst women and young people in Japan. Appleby and his colleagues observe that the regular misreporting of suicide rates by the media and in social media was in itself risky. One major risk is copycat self-destruction. They make a plea for responsible journalism and responsibility by users of social when commentating about suicide rates.

However, there is a wider issue regarding responsibility. The constant commentary about 'mental health problems' and new mental health initiatives, the popularisation of celebrity and Royal 'confessions' about psychological suffering, the growth in the genre of psychological self-help materials (in the form of books, TV documentaries and talk shows, and digital programmes), and in professionalised help (in the form of psychotherapy), is also risky. One major risk is more mental-healthism.

Appleby, in an opinion piece in the British Medical Journal, does call for a higher level of responsibility. Implicitly he is supporting the idea of a saner society to tackle psychological suffering and suicide:

> We need to rediscover the values that unite us and the benefits of mutual support. We need to reassure ourselves that there is a way out of this crisis and a better, fairer, more compassionate society at the end of it.
>
> (Appleby, 2021)

It wasn't only suicide that defied expectations throughout the COVID-19 pandemic. According to the Office for National Statistics (2022) homicide in England and Wales in the year ending March 2021, there were 594 homicide victims. Nearly 600 deaths cause much suffering (Morrall, 2000).

There are nearly half-a-million killings per year registered are homicides globally (United Nations Office on Drugs and Crime, 2019). Any death from homicide leaves multiple secondary victims, the family, friends, and close associates of the primary victims). Communities can endure tertiary victimhood especially when killings take place within their locality. However, the number of homicides in that year in England and Wales was a significant reduction from the previous year (79 fewer), and the lowest number and the lowest number for many years.

On the other hand, the rate of homicides in the USA during the first year of the pandemic went in the other direction to that of England and Wales. The number of homicides there increased by 30% (Houry *et al.*, 2022). The increase occurred in both cities and rural areas and in states with both Republican and Democratic voting majorities. There were many factors conjectured to have led to this rise. Some of these factors are particular to countries such as the USA but not as relevant to England and Wales. The proliferation of guns reduced public trust in the police, and the emotional distress associated with the pandemic are suggested as causes for this increase in the USA (Mekouar, 2022). Public trust, however, although traditionally not a major public issue in the UK except for certain sections of the population and in Northern Ireland, it has become more so in the rest of the UK since the pandemic (Wistrich, 2022). Although the homicide level dropped when COVID-19 lockdowns were introduced in the UK, it went back to pre-pandemic levels afterwards (ONS, 2022).

Common considerations connecting England and Wales to the USA during the pandemic, but which produced a difference in homicide trajectories, were employment and economic uncertainty, and a more severe structural separation in society between ethnic groups. Moreover, counties with existing high levels of gun ownership as well as poverty levels at the time of the pandemic also experienced the greatest increases in homicide (Houry *et al.*, 2022).

Medicalisation and Healthism

The notion of mental-healthism owes its conceptual heritage to a series of ideas contained in the social literature that has over decades developed critiques relating to psychological suffering. It has associations with concepts such as 'psycho-healthism' (Morrall, 2009) and the 'psy-complex' (Rose, 1985), as well as with theories examining how human 'civilisation' has manufactured madness (Foucault, 1961) and managed those deemed mad (Scull, 2015).

However, it is political economist Robert Crawford's (1980) idea of 'healthism' that provides the core intellectual underpinning of mental-healthism. The idea of healthism also has a heritage. It arose from critiques of the position and practices of the medical profession in society. These critiques posited that the rise in the status and influence of the medical profession had the effect of unduly 'medicalising' aspects of human performance that had beforehand been accepted as either normal, and therefore not requiring interventions of any kind, or abnormal but categorised in non-medical ways such as criminal, eccentric, foreignness, or the outcome of God's or the Devil's outrage.

The meaning of medicalisation, therefore, is more and more behaviours, thoughts, and emotions, have steadily come under the influence of the profession of medicine and this encompasses a wide and continually expanding rage of both somatic and psychological states (Conrad and Schneider, 1980). The medicalisation of everyday life in the West, having been progressing slowly for centuries, is now rampant. Moreover, Medicalisation is rampaging across global society and cyber society and is doing so even more successfully due to the encompassing of former epistemological enemies. Novel syndromes, maladies, and disorders are discovered or invented regularly. A huge variety of personal and social phenomena is now administrated by the medical expansionist enterprise despite the alleviating intervention of the internal censure. Body size and appearance, eating habits (for example, snacking and eating late in the day) and food constituents (for example, levels of fat, salt, and sugar), old age, social deviancy (for example, criminality and political unorthodoxy), not seeping enough and too much sleep, alcohol intake, tiredness, miserableness, excessive excitement, stressfulness, under-activeness and over-activeness,

Contributing to medicalisation is a wide and continually expanding range of both somatic and psychological purported remedies from disciplines allied and antagonistic to the power of the medical profession. Allies include pharmacy, and antagonists include psychology. However, as is exemplified by 'complementary' therapy, some of these disciplines have at times an allegiance to the medical profession, and thereby further the process of medicalisation, while at other times are antagonistic because they foster alternative epistemologies and practices.

Sociologist Irving Zola (Illich *et al.*, 1977), a foremost proponent of the idea of medicalisation views medicalisation as specialist social control whereby the State empowers the medical profession to handle those 'deviant' behaviours, thoughts, and emotions that are regarded as actually potentially destabilising the extant social hierarchy. Zola proclaimed medicalisation to have undermined human liberty. Hence, to achieve liberation, the de-medicalisation of society was necessary.

For philosopher and Catholic priest Ivan Illich (1975), the medical profession is extremely damaging to both people and society. Paradoxically, medicalisation has put both the well-being of individuals and the function of societal systems in jeopardy due to iatrogenesis, that is, the harm that is caused by the influence and interventions of medical practitioners. Medical influence and interventions, argues Illich, are such a cause of morbidity and mortality it can be viewed as one of the most rapidly spreading epidemics of modern times. Illich wrote his critique of the medical profession in the 1970s, Today, medicalisation is as if an infectious pandemic has spread as medical authority over everyday life ascended unabated by any would-be antidote. Notwithstanding countervailing forces (including the ascendence of scepticism about medical effectiveness and cynicism about expertise including science, along with the antagonists), the power of the medical profession is advancing. Although medical authority today is enhanced through the invention and application of increasingly sophisticated technology. Such technology covers diagnostic equipment (for example, computed tomography and magnetic resonance imaging scans), novel pharmaceutical products (notably mRNA vaccines), gene therapies, and surgical robotics.

Illich considered three forms of iatrogenesis. First, is 'clinical iatrogenesis'. This is the most obvious and understandable negative consequence of medicalisation, the declared and undeclared somatic and psychological side-effects to patients from the medication they receive or from surgery they undergo, mistakes in their care and treatment, and from hospital infections. Second, is 'social iatrogenesis' whereby the whole of society becomes dependent on medical products and medical knowledge medical profession. People become addicted not just to medicines but to medical discourse. That discourse becomes embedded in human culture. This effect is what Illich describes as 'cultural iatrogenesis'. Clinical iatrogenesis and social iatrogenesis lead to such entrenchment of medical authority in human culture that the individual loses his/her ability to make autonomous judgements. Medical practitioners have taken over from religious leaders (remembering that Illich was a priest) conferring advice and reinterpreting cultural norms and values redolent of biblical or Koranic instruction. Not only are individuals unable to make personal decisions about their lives, their experiences of physical pain, psychological suffering, and demise and death as inescapable elements of existence are nullified or mollified. Therefore, for Illich humans have become separated from their own humanness, from nature, and from reality. For humans to regain control of their humanness Illich advocates the de-professionalisation of all professions.

However, the concept of medicalisation has become accepted as having an element of legitimacy by the medical profession with articles by both social scientists and medical practitioners published on the subject in prestigious medical journals (for example, Le Fanu, 2018; Rose 2007). In part, this acceptance is because medicalisation is palpable in everyday medical practice. Medical practitioners face incessant pressure from pharmaceutical companies and the purveyors of a host of other purported therapeutic products along with petitions from their patients for pills and portions when advice or no intervention at all would suffice. Moreover, psychologist and sociologist Joan Busfield in her review of the term counsels that it should be applied judiciously:

> [Medicalisation] should not be read as necessarily assuming either passive patients, or empire-building by medical professionals, whether in alliance with corporations or not, though the activities of doctors and their enthusiasm for new technologies can contribute to instances of medicalisation. Nor should it be read as making some generalised attack on medicine, which can and often does ameliorate individuals' health problems.
>
> (Busfield, 2017, p.771)

The medical gaze, especially when focusing through biomedical and pharmaceutical lenses, is myopic. Healthism has far more scope than that of the medical gaze but is equally myopic. That is, both medicalisation and healthism situate the problem of health and ill-health at the level of the individual. Sources and solutions of health and ill-health are formulated also at that level. Both inherently diminish or disregard the social (economic and political) contexts (causes and cures) of much if not all of healthiness and ill-healthiness. Healthism more so than medicalisation, however, positions health as a 'super value' personifying the person as pivotal in the production of her/his well-being and unwellness (Crawford, 1980). Those fostering healthism, whom Crawford refers to as 'healthists', may concede that factors external to the individual influence personal choice (for example, the tobacco and food industry's advertising of products manifestly harmful to health), but determine that personal preference perseveres not matter the outside pressures. In other words, the individual has the responsibility for achieving and maintaining well-being and avoiding or assuaging unwellness. Moreover, health has become commodified. Healthism is part of the consumer culture with copious commodities supplied by drug companies, fashion industries, and sports/fitness enterprises. The commodity of 'mental health' is serviced by psychiatrists, psychologists, psychotherapists, and the gurus of self-help commerce.

The public issue of health has been refashioned as a private problem through healthism. Healthism pardons the primary perpetrations of physical illness and mental-healthism masks the main momenta for psychological suffering. These perpetrations and momenta include violence, inequality, selfishness, insecurity, and stupidity. A society that is sick is thereby sustained because sickness is seen to be sited elsewhere.

It is worth noting that mental-healthism, as with societal insanities and disasters, may not be wholly harmful to society or people. For example, although civilisations and empires may be undermined if not obliterated in the aftermath of a disaster, social progress is an outcome of previous major catastrophes such as the medieval plagues (Spinney, 2018). If the 'plague' of loneliness is reimagined as 'aloneness' then it may be experienced as a life choice which enables self-reliance (Kraybill, 2020). It is worth repeating that the concept of mental-healthism is not meant to minimise madness but mediate its meaning. Psychological suffering for some is patently profound but for others is either self-construed or professionally constructed as such notwithstanding the seemingly speciousness of their travails.

Mental Health Meanings

Psychologist Lucy Foulkes in her book titled 'Losing Our Minds: What Mental Illness Really Is and What It Isn't' (2021) asks how can 'normal' suffering be distinguished from 'abnormal'? She argues that the muddled thinking that surrounds attempts to understand these two fundamental concepts concerning human performance has had serious, sometimes life-changing if not life-ending consequences. Foulkes also flags the problem of mental-healthism (she doesn't use that term) when she by asking whether the lack of clarity about what is normal and what is abnormal is contributing to the rise in reporting of 'mental health problems' and the psychiatric diagnoses of mental disorder. For Foulkes, miserableness and worrying are part of the human condition. Unhappiness and angst do not equate to unwellness, and certainly should not attract a diagnosis of mental disorder. Foulkes accepts that mental illness exists but claims that its meaning is pervasively misunderstood. For her many aspects of normal psychological suffering becomes classified as mental disorder. She also suggests that heightened attention to psychological suffering is accompanied by a drive for instant fixing. The drive for immediate mending of the mind has become professionalised and commercialised with a host of professed experts offering advice for a price through self-help programmes and literature, a plethora of therapies and an enormous hike in both over-the-counter and prescribed medication.

In public discourse and in traditional and online media common emotional, behavioural, and cognitive difficulties and disparities are commonly described using medical terms for uncommon forms of psychological suffering. Disagreements over the meaning of mental disorder amongst and between professional and academic groupings make matters more mystifying. Some psychiatrists, psychologists, and sociologists, go so far as to claim all mental disorder is mythical. There is also the 'celebrity confessional syndrome' whereby the famous publicly announce their experience of psychological suffering and/or mental disorder diagnosis (Morrall, 2017).

For Foulkes, the attention and resources given to normal psychological suffering divert attention from those with a genuine mental disorder. This points to the paradox of contending, on the one hand, that too much normality is classified as an abnormality and, on the other hand, that much of abnormal psychological suffering is not being recognised.

> Therein lies the strange paradox we face right now, with all [mental] disorders. We are overdiagnosing mental illness, coating too many types of distress in psychiatric language, but the confusing thing is that we are also underdiagnosing some cases. So much devastating mental illness is still going unmanaged and untreated.
>
> (Foulkes, 2021, p.174)

Foulkes exposes another inconsistency when there is at the same time a rising awareness of suffering and her awareness that this leads to indiscriminate and inappropriate tagging of everyday mental messiness. Furthermore, Foulkes questions whether both or either the purported mental health crisis prior to the COVID-19 pandemic and the declared mental health crisis of the pandemic really should be considered as such.

> What is it about this generation, about today's society….that could mean we're suddenly in a collective psychiatric crisis?
>
> (Foulkes, 2021, p.11)

Much reporting of 'mental health problems' relies on the self-reporting of symptoms in questionnaires and interviews that are not necessarily designed to be robust measures of disorder or are composed by non-specialists to satisfy commercial and media needs. One or two symptoms, particularly if mild, do not equate to mental disorder but there is a tendency to conflate this distinction. Moreover, mental health awareness and anti-stigma campaigns may be contributing to the problem.

Reflecting on data from Europe, North America, South America, Asia, and Australia, Foulkes concludes that the increase in (genuine) mental disorder overall is small especially when compared to reports of crises. Most people who experience highly stressful events do not develop PTSD. Bereavement is not a disorder. Before the COVID-19 pandemic, indications of serious mental disorder, however, had increased significantly. These include self-harm in England and global rates of suicide. For Foulkes, the reasons for the rise in self-harm and suicide are as yet not known. Moreover, the pandemic altered these patterns.

So, psychological suffering as a subject has contending comprehensions. However, the dominance of the biomedical model and the rise of scientific modes of exploration and explanation based on empiricism in psychiatry along with physical methods of treatment (mainly pharmaceuticals) dominate in contemporary psychiatry. Foulkes comments on the deficits of this paradigm:

> Research so far has told us there is not an individual gene that codes for any specific mental illness. There is no 'bipolar disorder gene' or 'bulimia gene'. Instead, mental disorders are *polygenic*: hundreds and possibly even thousands of different genes play a role....
>
> (Foulkes, 2021, p.71)

Some genes may predispose some people to suffer some forms of psychological suffering and some of this suffering may susceptible to psychiatric classification. In most cases, these genetic predispositions need to be 'activated' by psychological or societal precipitating factors such as bad parenting and child abuse, stressful life events (for example, divorce, taking examinations, the death of a loved one), poverty, inequality, and physical disability.

For most mental disorders there is no established genetic causation or any sort of biological marker. Sophisticated microscopic and scanning technologies searching for neurological abnormalities linkable to mental disorder in the main do not resolve the cause-and-effect conundrum, nor the epistemological debating about the meaning of mental abnormality and normality. There is no scan or blood test that can diagnose any mental disorder. There is no one epistemological position that can uncontestably define ordinary and extraordinary psychological suffering or demarcate the two.

Foulkes takes the position that there is a spectrum of psychological suffering, and normalcy and pathology should not be confused. I take the position that normalcy and pathology may be unknowable, but some people are so troubled or troubling that they do need help but that help need not necessarily be medical, and in the long-term making society saner is more helpful (Morrall, 2017).

There is nuance regarding psychological suffering on top of the controversial application about applying medical labels to certain emotions, thoughts, and actions considered by psychiatry (arguably often with the encouragement of the State) to be pathological. Across a number of countries, negative emotions rose early on in the pandemic, only to fall after lockdowns started. As already mentioned, there is much evidence of psychological suffering through being separated from in-person social contact, loneliness, experiencing economic uncertainty, boredom, frustration, and managing childcare while also working. There is also evidence from countries such as the UK, New Zealand, Australia, India, South Africa, Ireland, the USA and Canada, that psychological suffering was assuaged when lockdowns were lifted. But paradoxically for some people happiness, optimism, contentment, and inspiration, increased, and sadness and fearfulness fell (Fabian *et al.*, 2020; Foa *et al.*, 2020).

Popular science writer Annaka Harris recalls the unresolved 'hard problem' of scientific research into consciousness. The unresolved 'hard problem' of scientific research into consciousness as the most important indicator of the existence of the 'self':

[W]e know that the idea of the self, as a concrete reality, is an illusion.
(Harris, 2019, p.94)

Harris observes that the main reason for the problem science has in fully understanding consciousness is because to date it does not have techniques or technologies that can provide insight into the relationship objective neurological matter has with subjective experience. She states bluntly that studying the brain merely reveals data about its physical properties not indubitable revelations about why humans, and possibly other forms of life, have awareness of their existence and can think about and give meaning to that awareness (Harris, 2019). Like so many scientific and social scientific concepts, finding a clear definition is a foregoing stumbling point. Studying any subject without an unambiguous and undisputed definition is likely to leave philosophers to wallow in the intellectual quagmire of conjecture, and researchers down blind alleys, into cul-de-sacs, or reporting misleading conclusions. The state of play in (not) understanding consciousness is highly significant for understanding human performance, especially those aspects that may become tagged as disordered. Put bluntly, if consciousness can't be comprehended then neither can psychological stability, and psychological suffering, let alone those parts of 'mental' human performance that become tagged as disordered.

Dexter Dias is a human rights lawyer, judge, and academic. He is also the author of a best-selling 'smart thinking' book titled *The Ten Types of Human: Who We Are and Who We Can Be* (Dias, 2018). His position on nature and nurture is not now novel. Both nature and nurture apply their influences on the emotional, cognitive, and behavioural tendencies of human performance. There is little left of the argument that one or the other wholly determines the entirety of human performance. Indeed, extreme social or biological determinism has left the intellectual stage, and although there remain a few die-hard determinists representing both social and biological hues are still presenting their scripts whether the plot is based on one version of Marxism whereby the mode of production is the governing socialising force, or seeing genes selfishly selecting the signifiers for who we are and what we can be.

Dias does, however, have an interesting twist on the dependence of nurture on nature when he suggests that social learning may be shaped by evolution. That is, millions of years of biological development in humans could have inculcated the content and processes of the societal norms and mores that then inculcate the performance of individuals. Dias is adamant that his view should not be misread as reinventing 'social Darwinism'. He is too late. It has already been resurrected. Myriad of academic and clinical disciplines have become the inheritors of social Darwinism, otherwise known as 'sociobiology' (Wilson, 1975). These include disciplines that purport to explain and thereafter rectify madness, notably evolutionary psychology, and evolutionary psychiatry.

The contention of the sociobiology thesis is that nature rather than nurture could explain all human traits from happiness to schizophrenia. For evolutionary psychologists (for example, Buss, 2014) and evolutionary psychiatrists (for example, Stevens and Price, 2000) all normal and abnormal human performance today stems from biological adaptations that have arisen far back in the history of humanity. While not all adaptations function fully for the benefit of survival and reproduction (the fundamental drivers of all forms of life), some that appear dysfunctional such as those aspects of human performance that secrete psychological suffering and may attract a psychiatric diagnosis have hidden advantages. For example, interludes of melancholy (possibly diagnosed as depression) can be functional in the sense that they might offer the opportunity to recover from a distressing event or think through complex problems by disengaging from everyday activities and responsibilities (Andrews and Thomson, 2009). Severe selfishness, high levels of manipulation, and a lack of remorse (possibly diagnosed as psychopathy or antisocial personality disorder) may have afforded an evolutionary advantage in dangerous times or when competition for mates was intense and may continue to offer an advantage in the world of corporate capitalism (Ene *et al.*, 2022). Evolutionary biologist and palaeontologist Stephen Jay Gould (1997) rails against these adaptations of Darwinian theory, describing them disparagingly as an 'attractive cult' that relies on post hoc theoretical suppositions rather than robust empirical evidence. Sociologist Andrew Scull (2007) adds to the criticism by arguing that not only is there a lack of empirical evidence to back up the ideas from evolutionary psychology and evolutionary psychiatry, but human history and its societal conditions is far too complex for any certainty to be established about the heritage and value of personal peculiarities. Scull also attacks the certainties presented by neuroscientists regarding the locus of madness, arguing that the complexities of human culture and neurophysiology cannot be simplified to the level of areas of the brain that light up when certain thoughts, emotions, and behaviours are expressed. For Scull, these simplistic biological reductionist conceptions are being used once again to assert psychiatry's status as a scientific discipline and thereby a suitable branch of the profession of medicine.

On the theme of the interconnectivity of nature and nurture Jolanta Burke, a psychologist specialising in the positive branch of her discipline, argues that genes at a molecular level influence and are influenced by the social environment. She reasons that if two people are brought up in the same social environment they may perform behaviourally, emotionally, and cognitively in very different ways because their biological propensities are different. But, in the example she provides, it may be that the two people have similar if not the same genomics (if they are identical twins) but that the social environment is imposing inconsistent pressures on them as individuals. Moreover, what Burke doesn't extricate from this example, however, is that both the 'nature' and the 'nurture' aspects of human disposition and experience are in such a complex and dynamic relationship as to make the linkage between them impossible to identify.

Notwithstanding that deficit in reasoning, Burke argues that the involvement of nature and nurture in human performance explains why some people are susceptible to significant readjustments to the way they think, feel, and act and others are not. She asserts, that there is no positive psychology intervention that will work for every person because due to genetic variation between individuals. Hence, from Burke's standpoint, it is not the ineffectiveness of such therapeutic inputs as positive psychology that may result in unhappy people remaining unhappy but the fault of their genes. Burke then qualifies this assertion by arguing that for those individuals who are endowed with what she refers to a 'genetic plasticity' (a more apposite descriptor for what it seems she means is 'brain plasticity'), then they could, especially with the assistance positive psychology's happiness tools, become happier. She does add, however, those with this plasticity can take advantage of social environments that encourage an increase in happiness. Burke sums up her position on nature and nurture as follows:

> [G]enetics does not determine who we are, even if it does play a significant role in our wellbeing. What also matters are the choices we make about….how we live our lives, which affect both our happiness and the happiness of the next generations.
>
> (Burke, 2021)

For sociologist Hilary Rose and neuroscientist Steven Rose (2016) the fixation on finding and fixing faults in the individual relies on what they describe as a 'crassly empiricist' epistemology. In the context of mental health crass empiricism refers to observing apparent abnormalities in genes, the brain and other parts of the neurological system, biochemical and gut micro-organism imbalance, and adverse inflammation. What is missing, argue Rose and Rose is not only robust theorising rather than assertions based on superficial surveillances of physiologies. Crucially, the elephant in the room in terms of intellectual aptitude and scientific method is the dynamic, multifarious, and immutable, influence of society on human performance – and *vice versa*.

There is, however, an evolutionary branch of sociology. That branch takes the lead from some of the founders of sociology who incorporated biology to a greater or lesser extent into their ideas about the formation and tribulations of society (Ho, 2023). Much of the 'new evolutionary sociology' reflects the need to recognise that dismissing biological influences, whether from the past or in the present, is intellectually unsustainable given the developments in the fields of genetics and neuroscience (Turner and Machalek, 2018). But the incorporation of biological ideas into sociological perspectives is very different to accepting the biological determinism that characterises sociobiology and its evolutionary offshoots in psychology and psychiatry.

For Nikolas Rose (2018) there are complex biological and societal connections participating in the cause of conditions that are medically described mental disorder and gives examples of schizophrenia and dementia. Just as some of the societal sources may have cultural ancestral origins, some of the biological determinants may have evolutionary foundations. Acting on these bygone causative components are the individual's extant societal and material circumstances. Regarding psychological suffering, material circumstances encompass both the physical environment hardships (ranging from poor housing to being bombed) and somatic misfortunes (including contracting a contagion). Moreover, Rose makes the point that all of these factors undergo cultural interpretations, including not being considered hardships, and 'psychological suffering' may also not be construed always as a negative experience. That said, Rose is an advocate for the marrying of sociological knowledge and biological evidence especially insights arising from neuroscience. He is also an advocate for psychiatrists and sociologists to combine and radicalise their relative political power (he observes that psychiatry has far more political power than his own discipline) to act as agents of social change. The social problems that are complicit in the causation of psychological suffering, especially severe forms that may lead to a mental disorder diagnosis, are presently not tackled in any effective way by psychiatry, psychotherapy, and psychology. This is due largely to the concentration of these disciplines on finding and fixing faults in the individual rather than fixing the faults in society that have already been found.

Significantly, Rose (2018) raises the issue of whether there is so much pathological psychological suffering and mental disorder as those who declare that there is an epidemic (and possibly a pandemic) in pathological states of mind. Rose challenges another metaphor employed by those proclaiming that psychological suffering has spread and intensified (whether or not medicalised) is only 'the tip of the iceberg'. The suggestion is that large numbers of people may be suffering psychologically in silence, or if not in silently then they are not receiving any or sufficient support. For Rose, society may be suffering from a spread and intensification of 'psychiatrisation'. That is, more and more states of mind have become medicalised as misfortunes in need of modification or abolition. Moreover, the psychiatrisation of society is most evident in Western countries but has been disseminated to undeveloped and developing countries.

The term 'psychiatrisation' implies it is psychiatry that is responsible for the contagion of conditions diagnosed as mental disorder. However, psychiatry is only one profession proliferating mental-healthism. Psychiatrisation and mental-healthism are societal contagions in the sense that once they 'infect' society they 'contaminate' more and more aspects of human performance. The concept of mental-healthism encompasses far more than those aspects of human performance that become diagnosed as mental disorder, and is aided by those disciplines that share a common epistemology and common practices with psychiatry no matter that they may be competing with their medical colleagues for epistemological occupational dominance. For the most part, psychiatry, psychotherapy, and psychology, share fundamental occupational philosophical approaches that are reified as finding and fixing faults in the individual and doing so based on empirical evidence. Their practices have commonality due to the focus on the individual. It is the individual who is examined, diagnosed (al-be-it using a profession-specific diagnostic schema or only informally), and to whom remedies are offered whether these are in the form of drugs or dialogue. Psychiatry differs here because it has the legal right, in certain circumstances, to enforce a treatment as well as incarceration. There are exceptions, with some practitioners from these disciplines rejecting individuation, and/or medicalisation. For these practitioners, there is an awareness that the culprit causing psychological suffering can be, and often is, society. They may also both drugs and dialogue of causing more harm than good because apart from side-effects from pharmaceuticals and the dubious effectiveness of some psychotherapies, treating the individual diverts attention from solving societal sources of psychological suffering (Morrall, 2017).

The worldwide rise in incidences of diagnosed mental disorders has the knock-on effect of escalating the use of health services. Some of this use is patently necessary. Those people experiencing a crisis in their mental health undoubtedly need help. But the process of psychiatrisation pulls into its sphere of sway many who would otherwise cope without medical input. There is then a growing burden to finance and staff these services. This burden is particularly severe for low-middle-income countries (Beeker *et al.*, 2021). Therefore, psychiatrisation rather than solving a problem in society (that is, poor mental health) becomes a problem for society. Psychiatrisation by boosting medical interventions aimed at the individual means depoliticising such social problems as inequality and violence.

Rose makes another apposite when he questions the logical inconsistency of psychiatry with its allegiance to biological understandings and the rise in diagnosed mental disorder, let alone the possible hidden numbers hidden in the underwater section of the 'iceberg'. Surely, he reasons, it is unreasonable to assume the biological makeup of humans has given the usual slow pace of evolution, radically changed, and done so within at most over a couple of hundred years to produce a mountain of mental disorder. The more reasoned cause of either undisputable and severe psychological suffering and/or psychiatrisation (and mental-healthism) is society.

If there really are scourges of, for example, miserableness and worrying then it is because of there are scourges of loneliness, interpersonal and inter-nation brutalities, huge divisions in wealth, employment uncertainty, rampant self-indulgence, and an ever-expanding mental health industry ever ready to offer or even impose its nomenclature and amenities. It is not because the human genome, the brain and linked neurological sub-systems, or the endocrine and immune systems, have in the space of a few generations become defective in millions of people. Nor has the mind, whether considered separate from the brain or merely the result of fortuitous synaptic connectivity, relatively suddenly become pathologically spoiled. On the other hand, society has mutated markedly over the same time. But what has also mutated markedly is the influence of the profession of medicine, big pharma, and all of the disciplines delivering their wares to the psychologically weary and unwary. Hence, certain characteristics of contemporary society could have inflicted a significant negative impression on the body and mind.

Rose (2018) concludes it is more complicated than blaming one societal system for all psychological suffering. To do so is to indulge in similar simplistic reasoning that has led to not referring to society when coming to conclusions about the characteristics of and cure for human ails whether psychological or physical. The issue of complexity is addressed well by medical practitioner and strident critic of big pharma and bad science, Ben Goldacre's (2015 book titled *I Think You'll Find It's a Bit More Complicated Than That* is relevant in this context. To understand mental health demands complex thinking and not thinking that is partisan). Regarding the diagnosis of mental disorder, where this medical ascription has legitimacy based on the seriousness of the distress, the relevance of societal circumstances is recognised by most neuroscientists and geneticists (Rose and Abi-Rached, 2013). Although the impact of society on the psyche may be incorporated into the underlying premises of biological investigation, it's impact on how they conduct research and what then is recommended regarding changing society is limited or omitted.

So, some positions can be taken about human performance founded on the robust theorising and empirical research that is presently available and generally agreed. Evolution has two fundamental biological drives for all life. These are to survive and reproduce. These drives and their derivatives are passed on through the generations genetically. Genes interact with other aspects of biology (for example, biochemicals and bacteria) and the physical environment. Added to the biological and physical environment interplay in humans and in other cognisant and sociable animals is the influence of consciousness and culture. In non-humans the presence, and if present the impact of consciousness and culture remains, debatable. It may be that such notions as consciousness and culture are inappropriate appellants for non-humans, perhaps exemplifying anthropomorphism imperialism and anthropocentrism rather than valid complementary qualities for humans and animals. The (conscious and cognitive) mind and the (material) brain are inseparable. If the position is taken that the workings of the former is considered only as the outcome of the workings of the latter, then the reverse is also a reasonable position. That is, the brain works the mind, and the mind works the brain. Both have plasticity, the mind abstractly and the brain concretely. Contributing considerably to this inconsistent concoction of biological and psychological stimuli are those supplied by society. Due to the volatile interplay of these biological, psychological, and societal, incitements, the performance of human emotions, thinking, and behaviour, contain consistencies and inconsistencies. Human performance is thereby replete with paradox, examples of which are pusillanimity and perseverance, and solidity and suffering. It's complicated.

Journalist Susannah Cahalan (2020), who had a neurological disorder misdiagnosed repeatedly as a mental disorder, has written about the lack of robust knowledge in psychiatry. For much of medical practice meant to address madness operates more on faith than certainty. Her personal insights through experience as a patient and subsequent investigation as a journalist into how some conceptualisations of mental disorder and critiques of psychiatric practice have been built on flawed research adds to the body of opinion that psychiatric prevention and cure for virtually all its medicalised madness has failed.

Psychiatrist Joanna Moncrieff is critical of her profession for increasing reliance on biological explanations for psychological suffering and on pharmaceuticals as the mainstay of treatment. A major criticism levelled at both her profession and the pharmaceutical industry by Moncrieff concerns the traditional view that the biochemical serotonin. Serotonin is a key neurotransmitter. It has multiple roles in the body responsible including moderating mood, and memory. It has been a major factor in supporting psychiatry's and the pharmaceutical industry's belief in biology. A low level of serotonin concentrations or activity is supposed to be associable with depression. Therefore, drugs altering the way serotonin operates have been designed, manufactured, and prescribed in their billions. But research by Moncrieff and her colleagues leads them to conclude that there is no hard evidence to support a link between serotonin and depression (Moncrieff *et al.*, 2022). Some serotonin altering drugs to seem to have a slight antidepressant effect accepts Moncrieff and her colleagues. However, these may only work a little better than does the placebo effect.

For Moncrieff (2020), not only antidepressants but all psychiatric drugs do not have the effect professed by their manufacturers and prescribers. They do not cure or even effectively ameliorate any mental disorder. They may dampen some symptoms – and so do inert pills – but at the cost of increasing suffering from side effects, some of which are so serious that they undermine an individual's ability to perform everyday activities. Hence, the side effects produce similar outcomes in terms of living normally as whatever condition it is they are supposed to remedy. Worse still is that they are difficult to be weaned off because doing so may produce other side effects and ones that may be just as severe as those caused by taking the drugs. Psychiatry's reliance on chemicals to impede or end emotional distress, argues Moncrieff, is the wrong approach.

Anthropologist and psychotherapist James Davies (2013) is also a critic of the psychiatry's reliance on pharmaceuticals for similar reasons to those of Moncrieff and her colleagues. However, for Davies, it is not only that psychiatric drugs do more harm than good but the whole of the psychiatric profession. Psychiatry, Davies proposes, is 'cracked' because it has allowed itself to be drawn into an unethical business approach whereby huge profits are made from the selling of harmful drugs.

The adherence by psychiatry to pharmaceutical interventions based on a biological model of madness does not in the main benefit their patients but themselves. Elevated professional status is the main benefit for psychiatry from propounding biology as the basis for myriad of psychological affectations most of which are spuriously designated as disorder. The biological model allows psychiatrists to claim epistemological parity with their colleagues in all the other sub-divisions of medicine. The biological allows the pharmaceutical companies to claim therapeutic legitimacy for the promotion of drugs as one if not the only solution for the ready-made and ever-expanding inventory of mental disorders.

According to critics of psychiatry's biology and drug dependency such as Davies and Moncrieff, much of the claimed relevancy and efficacy of these psycho-pharmaceuticals is founded on the misrepresentation of research results, short-term analysis of data when a longer review of the evidence might indicate inefficacy or adverse side-effects, the discarding of results that show no positive effects, and mass marketing targeting both the public and professionals. Moreover, as public health scholar China Mills (2014) notes, more and more non-Western nations are succumbing to the 'colonisation' of Western-style psychiatric conceptualisations of and cures for psychological suffering.

The proliferation of Western psychiatry globally along with the expansion of related disciplines and the institutional set-ups needed to deliver their practices also proliferates mental-healthism. More mental health professionals and mental health services means the 'uncovering' of more mental disorders and thereby more people become patients or clients. There is an important caveat to the claim of psychiatric global colonisation. Many countries in the world no not have many mental health professionals and if they have any formal mental health service it may be drastically inadequate due to under-funding, deficient infrastructure. The use of psychiatric drugs may also be limited because of cost. This is especially so in low-income countries. But as Dévora Kestel, Director of the Department of Mental Health and Substance Use at the World Health Organisation points out, far from the world being 'psychiatrised', there is a lack of provision in most countries:

> Most societies and most health and social systems neglect mental health and do not provide the care and support people need and deserve. The result is that millions of people around the world suffer in silence, experience human rights violations or are negatively affected in their daily lives.
> (Kestel quoted in World Health Organisation, 2022b, p.vii)

In the World Health Organisation's report containing Kestel's comment, it is stated that one in eight people globally suffer from a mental disorder, and about half of the global population lives in countries where there is only one psychiatrist for approximately 2,000,000 people. The report goes on to state that the availability of what it claims are 'essential' psychotropic drugs is limited, especially the case in low-income countries, and that most people with a diagnosed mental disorder do not get any (formal) treatment. The reasons offered in the report for the under-staffing, under-resourcing, and under-treating for people with a diagnosed (or diagnosable) mental disorder include the cost of treatment and inaccessibility of services where they do exist, the prioritising of other health problems, an absence of research into mental disorder, and of political will and governance and dedicated funding, Regarding the latter, the report states that on average, governments dedicate less than 2% of their budget on health care to mental health.

Furthermore, stigma continues to be attributed to a diagnosis of mental disorder throughout the world, but in poorer countries this may be more marked. What the World Health Organisation in the above report is does not highlight is the conscious choice people may be making to cope with psychological suffering rather than seek formal help or that it may be culturally acceptable to 'suffer in silence'. Help for unwelcome mental distress as packaged by Western psychiatry and its professional and corporate confederates may also unacceptable be well as unnecessary.

Drugs remain the most used psychiatric treatment in the Western countries. However, having made enormous profits from the selling of psychotropic drugs, towards the end of the first decade of the 20th century, the pharmaceutic industry stopped investing in these products. Particularly noticeable has been the de-investment in the research and development of new drugs depression, bipolar disorder, schizophrenia. The pharmaceutical industry's loss of interest has been framed as a crisis for both psychiatry. It has also been described as a crisis for patients by those who proclaim that psychotropic drugs have been successful in lessoning the severity of symptoms, and in allowing patients to live as normal a life as their moderated condition will allow.

Steven Hyman, a psychiatrist, and researcher specialising in stem cell and regenerative biology, is aware of the complexities involved in linking biological factors, mental disorders, and drug treatments. He is aware that these complex links have yet to be unravelled to the point that specific biomarkers can be attributed to specific mental disorders. He is aware of the failings of the extant psychiatric pharmacopoeia in terms of their efficacy and side-effects. He also makes the diagnosis of a crisis in psychiatric drug research and development. That does not stop him from arguing that even the existing drugs have been 'great blessing to many patients and their families' (Hyman, 2013). But for Robert Whitaker (2019) the crisis in psychiatry goes far beyond that concerning the availability of its pharmaceutical treatments. The crisis is one that concerns the legitimacy of psychiatry as a profession and the authenticity of the array of mental disorders it has made available, based on failed promises, flawed science, and the false construction of faults in the individual.

The pharmaceutical industry has drawn back its involvement in producing psychiatric drugs for a combination of reasons. Many of the original drugs used by psychiatry are out-of-patent, making their generic reproductions cheaper. More profitable (and efficacious) drug markets to exploit have surfaced, including drugs to combat cancer and mass vaccination. Alternative and cheaper offerings for the alleviation of distressful mental states such as cognitive behavioural therapy have ascended. These reasons are supplementary to that of the moot merit of medication for treating diagnosed mental disorders let alone 'normal' (and undiagnosed) apprehension and unhappiness. At the same time, psychiatry has been struggling to exploit the expanding amount of scientific knowledge being gained about the cellular and molecular foundations of life, and to utilise gene editing technology.

Davies (2022) blames capitalism for what he claims are the dubious ideas and actions of pharmaceutical companies and psychiatry. He expressly accuses psychiatrists of being in league with, and the lackey of, 'neo-liberal' corporate capitalists. The neoliberal doctrine is a mixture of lauding individualism, disparaging the collective, drastically reducing the State's role in the economy and contribution to housing, health, social care, education, and welfare support, advocating self-responsibility and self-regulation, and offering countless commodities to sustain rabid consumption. Psychiatry partakes in the delivery of this doctrine by commodifying madness and expanding its range of commodities through the process of medicalising not only madness but normality. Davies argues that the medicalisation of psychological suffering is clearly not working. But then how can he also argue that psychiatry is successful is State sponsored undertaking to sedate the population?

Sociologist Bruce Cohen (2016) also blames capitalism. What Cohen offers is a Marxist analysis of psychiatry that focuses on its historical association with the State and its willing incorporation into what he regards as a mode of production that although riddled with subtle inequities in essence sponsors a binary division. This binary division is founded on finance. This is a straightforward explication of Marxist economics whereby the structure of society is split into one small section made-up of an elite who controls and benefit from economic resources and the rest of the population who have little if any control and derive few benefits from these resources. Psychiatry participates in this inequitable bifurcation of society. It is in league with the politically powerful and those whose power is derived from the ownership of large national and transnational corporations. Control is exercised in the main through socialising the exploited majority into accepting that the ways in which politics and business operate are economically and morally legitimate and that the social hierarchy is necessary to ensure financial and ethical sustainability. As part of the socialisation process, the message that the *status quo* means 'safety' in the sense that conversion to any other way of managing society (particularly its economy) would herald uncontainable and devastating social crises. In the propaganda of the powerful are allusions to disastrous historical events. One of those allusions is what happened when Tsarist Russia fell to the Bolsheviks in the October Revolution of 1917 and millions of Russians were later executed by fellow Russians or incarcerated in Siberian Gulags. Another is what happened in China after Mao Zedong proclaimed the establishment of The People's Republic of China in October 1949 and the subsequent millions of deaths from war, famine, and the 'Cultural Revolutions' pogroms. A third is what happened because of the rise and fall of German and Italian fascism in the mid-20th century. Furthermore, adopting this uncomplicated Marxist perspective the indoctrinating subtleties disseminated by those with political and economic encompass the message that is only the variation of capitalism in existence presently that can deliver innovative knowledge and technologies so solve such social crises as the COVID-19 pandemic, the war in Ukraine, and madness.

But it is more complicated than that. It is also more contradictory. For example, economist Constantinos Alexiou (2021) claims to have spotted a complicated contradiction concerning COVID-19 and capitalism. The pandemic, he suggests, has exposed the Achille's heel of capitalism. The weakness he identifies is in how in 2020 the global elites and the capitalist economic system, faced what he states was the 'multifaceted crisis' of the pandemic, and failed. Capitalism itself fell into the worse crisis in its history, unable to adjust to the new circumstances of reduced economic activity, failing business, and recession, let alone supply health systems and health and emergency workers with adequate resources and personal protective equipment to save swathes of people from the debility and death. Alexiou's prediction of the curtailing of induced by the pandemic was published in May 2021. Today capitalism, with all of its complexities and contradictions, continues. It has not failed, at least not yet. Moreover, contagions, conflicts, and the plethora of supposed psychiatric sicknesses persist in the nourishing market economy. Money is still made from mayhem and maladies. Cohen, a persistent critic of capitalism, inconsistently points to a major reason why this economic system persists and for the same reason why the power of psychiatry persists. The Cohen provides is 'hegemony'.

The ancient Greek term hegemony has been adopted by a host of radical social thinkers and activists to explain how political dominance is maintained in large part through a process of ideological indoctrination (Martin, 2022). Those adopting hegemony to analyse political power may use the insights gained to undermine the social control exercised by those in presently in power to install radical reform. Cohen joins a wide variety of academics and activists who have taken this approach. These include the leader of the Bolshevik revolution in Russia Vladimir Lenin, Italian political philosopher Antonio Gramsci, educational philosopher Paulo Freire, cultural theorist Stuart Hall, linguist and philosopher Noam Chomsky, criminologist Jock Young, and another sociologist specialising in the study of madness Andrew Scull.

What is missing from Cohen's would-be revolutionary project are any specifics about how to help those who are presently suffering psychologically no matter that the causes of this suffering are societal. Furthermore, academics who critique and criticise social systems have a social responsibility, a moral duty, to contribute to specifying and then sorting a better system not merely sit on the sidelines if and when their desired changes have begun to transpire. That is activism to be ethical and effective requires a combination of intellectualism and pragmaticism.

But is not only oblique social control that occurs in psychiatric practice. Psychiatry in the past has utilised blatant and patently barbaric physical methods of treatment. The present use of chemicals by psychiatry as its main form of treatment is also easily understood as dampening deviations from what is construed as normal behaviours, thoughts, and emotions. However, Cohen cites certain exceptional situations to support his thesis that psychiatry is essentially an agency of hegemonic regulation on behalf of the powerful and to further its own power. For example, he refers to psychiatry's collusion with Nazis before and during the Second World War. Psychiatrists participated in atrocities including conducting cruel experiments and ruthless exterminations.

The denunciation of the whole of psychiatry past and present because of such barbarisms, however, is to embark on an unsustainable generalisation akin to denouncing the whole of the German population past and present for the conduct of the Nazis. Cohen's position is far more intellectually and empirically legitimate when focusing on the pervasive intricacies of psychiatric hegemony rather than infrequent incidents of barefaced barbarity.

Cohen also collaborates in contradiction of claiming that psychiatry serves well the interests of capitalism by controlling performances that are deemed by capitalists to be damaging to that economic system yet there is a substantial increase in the diagnosis of disorder. The upsurge in diagnoses has followed the same trajectory as the upsurge in psychiatric hegemonic power. But if psychiatry is participating in the capitalistic hegemonic social control, then neither are being very effective given that social deviancy in the form of medicalised madness is accelerating.

Moreover, for Cohen as it is for Davies it is the neoliberal form of capitalism that is outstandingly capable in its capacity to inculcate social control by selling self-responsibility and self-regulation as primary aspects of acceptable human performance. Focusing on the self as the locus of responsibility and regulation, along with the locus of causes and cures for irresponsible and unregulated emotions, thoughts, and behaviours, all fit with the tenets of contemporary capitalism and psychiatry. Joining psychiatry in this hegemonic task on behalf of neoliberal capitalism is psychopharmacology as well as psychotherapy and psychology. If Cohen is correct about the power of psychiatry's role in helping neoliberal hegemony, then it has been a calamitous failure if measured by how many people are now categorised as deviating from neoliberal norms and pathologised as mentally disordered. On the one hand, if psychiatry is operating only as another capitalist corporation (along with psychopharmacology, psychotherapy, and psychology) then it is exceedingly successful if measured by its market spread.

Davies (2022) is caught in a contradiction that complements Cohen's. He has two inconsistent strands to his criticism of capitalism. First, he argues that capitalism has caused a crisis in psychological suffering, but then argues that this is a contrived crisis created by capitalism. Davies concedes that sincere psychological suffering has increased, the cause of which for him has been the increase in the harmful effects of neoliberalism. Since the 1980s capitalism's neoliberal mutation began in the USA under the leadership of Ronald Reagan and in the UK under the leadership of Margaret Thatcher. Since then, it has spread its influence, mostly surreptitiously, to become the reigning political-economic theory globally (Metcalf, 2017). For Davies and Cohen neoliberal capitalism has also permitted psychiatry and the other 'psy' professions, and psychopharmacology, to innovate and disseminate more forms of medicalised madness and thereby more and more of their would-be remedies. Following the logic of Davies and Cohen contentions, the mental health crisis has formed a lucrative marketplace for the sale of psychiatric services, whether this crisis has authentic or bogue. But what neither do is to clearly demarcate the psychological suffering that occurs separately to that induced by neoliberalism capitalism, non-liberal capitalism, alternative political-economic setups, or other factors in society below those of overall structural arrangements. Nor are faulty features of an individual's psychological and biological constitution given the credibility they warrant in respect of possible factors in the causation of emotional distress. The trouble with fixating on neoliberal capitalism is the baby is being thrown out with the bathwater.

Raising the status of societal sources of mental muddles and misgivings should not be on the cost of displacing other causes that have legitimate supportive evidence. Dementia and general paralysis of the insane (neurosyphilis) are caused by biological pathology, are objectively diagnosable, and the latter is treatable pharmacologically and there is the potential for the former to be similarly correctable if only to a partial extent. That said, societal situations such as neoliberalism shape the formation, progress, and outcomes, of these and all other experiences of psychological suffering. In societies where economic expansionism is the predominating political mandate and commodification and consumerism its concomitant cultural values, and the involvement of the State in health and social care in minimalised, then research into and treatment for emotional distress with distinct non-societal dispositions may not be prioritised unless to do so will be profitable. Alternatively, the neoliberal economic imperative may capitalise on a market that is ripe to be expanded and exploited. This is because of the sanctification and centralisation of the self within that variant of capitalism. Consequently, psychological suffering succumbs to commodification and consumerism.

Psychiatrist Awais Aftab affirms the commitment of his discipline to biology but also, perhaps unwittingly, posits the very reason that this adherence to the framing of even psychological suffering that is medicalised is not only problematic but fallacious

> Most mental disorders are presumed by psychiatrists] to have a neurobiological basis even in cases in which this basis is poorly understood….. We still do not have fully satisfactory definitions of either disease or mental disorder, and I do not attempt to argue that the current conceptualizations are unproblematic.
>
> (Aftab, 2014)

Aftab cannot justifiably downplay that current conceptualisation of mental disorder are 'unproblematic' and that there are not only are some of these disorders poorly comprehended as well as definitional inaccuracy remains for mental disorder (as a physical disease). How can psychiatry have reached the point of compiling a tome of mental disorders that is the DSM, and how can then the plethora of physical and psychotherapeutic preparations be prescribed, without having its own practitioners first procuring an agreed meaning for mental disorder?

Aftab in the article in which the above quotation is taken is reviewing the contentions of fellow psychiatrist Thomas Szasz. Szasz exposed an elementary ambiguity in the claim of his biologically minded psychiatric colleagues. For Szasz (1961) mental 'illness' (or mental disorder or mental disease) is a myth because 'mental' is an abstract concept whereas 'illness' is only conceptually valid when there is an objectively identifiable physical pathological properties present. However, if as claimed by psychiatrists embedded in a biological epistemology, there are physical pathological properties present in a mental disorder then it is not a 'mental' disorder but a 'brain' (or neurological) disorder. Moreover, if physical pathology present then it is not any more the province of the psychiatric branch of the profession of medicine that should be involved by neurology. That is organically disordered, disordered, or ill brains or any other part of the neurological system can benefit from far more precise defining than, for example, schizophrenia and personality disorder, and thereby afforded treatments aimed at an identified target.

As Davies (2022) submits, neo-liberal capitalism generates the conditions for increasing psychological suffering and profitable depoliticised remedial interventions. For Davies, the present-day dominant global economic system has interfered more radically and pervasively with the traditional cultural and human values than had already occurred during earlier variations of capitalism. Furthermore, the undermining of community, cooperation, critical reasoning, compassion, and creativity, has had a dehumanising effect. There has been a neutering of humanity's 'vital energies'. These vital energies, for Davies, are required by humans in order to live authentically and civilise society. Davies comments that suffering is a necessary precondition for social change.

Davies does provide examples of circumstances during the COVID-19 pandemic that enhanced psychological solidity. He notes, as have others, that the air was cleaner especially during lockdowns because of the reduction in traffic on the roads, families spent more time together, and many workers were either given the choice or legally obliged to stay at home to work curtailed thereby avoiding have to commute, other workers were given financial support to stop working altogether thereby relieving the stress of working in alienating jobs, high street consumerism diminished (although it increased via the internet), and daily living overall became calmer. For Davies back to normal should not be the choice. But Davies does not stipulate specific epistemological and practical strategies indicating precisely how this should be achieved.

Summary

There is no biological or other medical justification for the creation and continued expansion of mental-healthism. There is no blood test, urine test, observation from any type of fully body or brain scan, or any other objective medical assessment akin to those associated with the diagnosis of cancer, heart disease, or infections such as COVID-19, to justify the majority of about 370 categories and hundreds more sub-categories contained in the fifth version of the DSM.

The concept of mental-healthism is in tune with the sentiments of Davies (2022), that all of the professions and corporations involved in managing mental health, that everyday human distress has been wrongly medicalised and pathologised. The signatories to cementing mental-healthism as a cultural normal are the advocates of a political and economic global system that preserves a host of societal insanities of inequality, violence, selfishness, insecurity, and stupidity, while lauding competitiveness, acquisitiveness, aggressiveness, deceitfulness, and powerfulness.

It is the insanities in society, not genetic defects, chemical imbalance, or cerebral irregularity, that cause sincere psychological suffering *and* the superimposing of synthetic suffering. Most ordinary psychological suffering is self-correcting and is therefore not in need of labelling and expert intervention. In the next chapter there is discussion on how most people cope and even hope no matter how trying or even terrible their circumstances,

Note

1 The idea of mental-healthism came from discussions between me, friends, and colleagues during (non-lockdown) periods of the COVID-19 pandemic. My thanks go especially to artist and ex-diplomat Keith Dunn, and psychotherapist Dr Greg Nolan.

References

Aftab A (2014) Mental Illness vs Brain Disorders: From Szasz to DSM-5. *Psychiatric Times*, 31(2). https://www.psychiatrictimes.com/view/mental-illness-vs-brain-disorders-szasz-dsm-5 [accessed 5th March, 2023]

Alexiou C (2021) Covid-19, Capitalism and Political Elites: The Real Threat to Humanity. *Human Geography* 14(2), pp.284–287.

Andrews P and Thomson A (2009) The Bright Side of Being Blue: Depression as an Adaptation for Analyzing Complex Problems. *Psychological Review*, 116(3), pp.620–654.

Appleby L (2021) What Has Been the Effect of Covid-19 on Suicide Rates? *British Medical Journal*, 372(834). https://www.bmj.com/content/372/bmj.n834 [accessed 25th July, 2022]

Appleby L, Richards N, Ibrahim S, Turnbull P, Rodway C and Kapur N (2021) Suicide in England in the COVID-19 Pandemic: Early Observational Data from Real Time Surveillance. *The Lancet*, 4(100110). https://www.thelancet.com/journals/lanepe/article/PIIS2666-7762(21)00087-9/fulltext [accessed 25th July, 2022]

Beeker T, Mills C, Bhugra D, Meerman S, Thoma S, Heinze M and von Peter S (2021) Psychiatrization of Society: A Conceptual Framework and Call for Transdisciplinary Research. https://www.ncbi.nlm.nih.gov/pmc/articles/PMC8211773/ [accessed 25th February, 2023]

Burke J (2021) Why Some People Find It Harder to be Happy. The Conversation, 26th November. https://theconversation.com/why-some-people-find-it-harder-to-be-happy-171692 [accessed 29th November, 2021]

Busfield J (2017) The Concept of Medicalisation Reassessed. *Sociology of Health and Illness*, 39(5), pp.759–774.

Buss D (2014) (fifth edition) *Evolutionary Psychology: The New Science of the Mind*. London: Routledge.

Cahalan S (2020) *The Great Pretender: The Undercover Mission that Change Our Understanding of Madness*. Edinburgh: Canongate.

Cohen B (2016) *Psychiatric Hegemony: A Marxist Theory of Mental Illness*. London: Palgrave Macmillan.

Conrad P and Schneider J (1980) *Deviance and Medicalisation: From Badness to Sickness*. St. Louis, MI: Mosby.

Conrad P and Slodden C (2013) *The Medicalization of Mental Disorder*. New York: Springer.

Crawford R (1980) Healthism and the Medicalization of Everyday Life. *International Journal of Health Services*, 3(10), pp.365–388.

Davies J (2013) *Cracked: Why Psychiatry is Doing More Harm Than Good*. London: Icon.

Davies J (2022) *Sedated: How Modern Capitalism Created Our Mental Health Crisis*. London: Atlantic.

Dias D (2018) *The Ten Types of Human: Who We Are and Who We Can Be*. London: Windmill.

Ene, I, Wong, K and Salali, G. (2022). Is It Good To Be Bad? An Evolutionary Analysis of Psychopathic Traits. *Evolutionary Human Sciences*, 4, pp.1–50. https://www.researchgate.net/publication/362632393_Is_it_good_to_be_bad_An_evolutionary_analysis_of_psychopathic_traits [accessed 23rd February, 2023]

Fabian M, Foa R and Gilbert S (2020) Wellbeing levels fell during the pandemic but improved under lockdown, data analysis shows. The Conversation, 30th July. https://theconversation.com/wellbeing-levels-fell-during-the-pandemic-but-improved-under-lockdown-data-analysis-shows-143367 [accessed 28th October, 2021]

Foa F, Gilbert S and Fabian M (2020) *COVID-19 and Subjective Well-Being: Separating the Effects of Lockdowns from the Pandemic*. Cambridge: Bennett Institute for Public Policy.

Foucault M (1961) *Folie et Déraison: Histoire de la folie à l'âge classique* [retitled in English as 'Madness and Civilization', New York, 1965]. Paris: Librarie Plon.

Foulkes L (2021) *Losing Our Minds: What Mental Illness Really Is and What It Isn't*. London: Bodley Head.

Goldacre B (2015) *I Think You'll Find It's a Bit More Complicated Than That*. London: Allen Lane.

Gould S J (1997) Darwinian Fundamentalism. *New York Review of Books* (June 12th), pp.34–37.

Harris A (2019) *Conscious: A Brief Guide to the Fundamental Mystery of the Mind*. New York: HarperCollins.

Ho W (2023) Returning Biology to Evolutionary Sociology: Reflections on the Conceptual Hiatuses of "New Evolutionary Sociology" as a Vantage Point. *Sociological Perspectives*, 66(1), pp.123–144.

Houry D, Simon T and Crosby A (2022) Firearm Homicide and Suicide During the COVID-19 Pandemic: Implications for Clinicians and Health Care Systems. https://jamanetwork.com/journals/jama/fullarticle/2792080 [accessed 25th July, 2022]

Hyman S (2013) Psychiatric Drug Development: Diagnosing a Crisis. *Cerebral*, 5(March–April). https://www.ncbi.nlm.nih.gov/pmc/articles/PMC3662213/. [accessed 1st March, 2023]

Illich I (1975) *Medical Nemesis: The Expropriation of Health*. London: Marian Boyars.

Illich I, Zola I and McKnight J (1977) *Disabling Professions*. London: Marion Boyars.

Kraybill O (2020) Moving From Loneliness to Aloneness. *Psychology Today*, June 30th. https://www.psychologytoday.com/us/blog/expressive-trauma-integration/202006/moving-loneliness-aloneness [accessed 26th November, 2020]

Laversuch C (2020) 'Bad busking is affecting our mental health' say city centre staff. York Press, 31st October. https://www.yorkpress.co.uk/news/18835888.bad-busking-affecting-mental-health-say-city-centre-staff/ [accessed 30th September, 2021]

Le Fanu J (2018) Mass Medicalisation is an Iatrogenic Catastrophe. *The British Medical Journal*, 361(k2794; June). https://www.bmj.com/content/361/bmj.k2794 [accessed 19th December, 2022]

Martin J (2022) *Hegemony*. Cambridge, UK: Polity Press.

Mekouar D (2022) Why Homicide Rates Spiked 30% During the Pandemic. https://www.homelandsecuritynewswire.com/dr20220202-why-homicide-rates-spiked-30-during-the-pandemic [accesses 28th March, 2023]

Metcalf S (2017). Neoliberalism: the idea that swallowed the world. *The Guardian*, 18th August. https://www.theguardian.com/news/2017/aug/18/neoliberalism-the-idea-that-changed-the-world [accessed 4th March, 2023]

Mills C (2014) *Decolonizing Global Mental Health: The Psychiatrization of the Majority World*. Abington-on-Thames: Routledge.

Moncrieff J (2020) *A Straight Talking Introduction to Psychiatric Drugs: The About How They Work and How to Come Off Them*. Monmouth: PCCS Books.

Moncrieff J, Cooper R, Stockmann T, Amendola S, Hengartner M and Horowitz M (2022) The Serotonin Theory of Depression: A Systematic Umbrella Review of The Evidence. *Molecular Psychiatry*, 20th July, pp.1–14. https://www.nature.com/articles/s41380-022-01661-0 [accessed 7th August, 2022]

Morrall P (2000) *Madness and Murder*. London: Whurr.

Morrall P (2009) *Sociology & Health: An Introduction*. London: Routledge.

Morrall P (2017) *Madness: Ideas about Insanity*. Abingdon, UK: Routledge.

National Institute for Health and Care Excellence (2020) Improving Access to Psychological Therapies (IAPT). https://www.nice.org.uk/about/what-we-do/our-programmes/nice-advice/iapt [accessed 17th April, 2020]

Office for National Statistics (2022) Homicide in England and Wales: Year Ending March 2021. Press Release, 10th February. https://www.ons.gov.uk/peoplepopulationandcommunity/crimeandjustice/articles/homicideinenglandandwales/yearendingmarch2021 [accessed 25th July, 2022]

Penninx B, Benro, Klein R and Vinkers C (2022) How COVID-19 Shaped Mental Health: from Infection to Pandemic Effects. *Nature Medicine*, 28(10), pp.2027–2037.

Pies R (2020) Is the Country Experiencing a Mental Health Pandemic? *Psychiatric Times*, 37(10). https://www.psychiatrictimes.com/view/are-we-really-witnessing-mental-health-pandemic [accessed 28th October, 2021]

Rose N (1985) *The Psychological Complex. Psychology, Politics and Society in England 1869–1939*. London: Routledge and Kegan Paul.

Rose N (2007) Beyond Medicalisation. *The Lancet*, 369(9562), pp.700–702.

Rose N (2018) *Our Psychiatric Future: The Politics of Mental Health*. Cambridge: Polity.

Rose N and Abi-Rached J (2013) *Neuro: The New Brain Sciences and the Management of the Mind*. Princeton, NJ: Princeton University Press.

Rose H and Rose S (2016) *Can Neuroscience Change Our Minds?* Cambridge: Polity.

Scull A (2007) Mind, Brain, Law and Culture – Book Reviews by Andrew Scull. *Brain*, 130, pp.585–591.

Scull A (2015) *Madness in Civilisation*. London: Thames and Hudson.

Soneson E, Puntis S, Chapman N, Mansfield K, Jones P and Fazel M (2022) Happier During Lockdown: A Descriptive Analysis of Self-Reported Wellbeing in 17,000 UK School Students During Covid-19 Lockdown. *European Child & Adolescent Psychiatry*, 17th February. https://link.springer.com/article/10.1007/s00787-021-01934-z [accessed 18th February, 2023]

Spinney L (2018) *Pale Rider: The Spanish Flu of 2018 and How It Changed the World*. London: Vintage.

Stevens A and Price J (2000) (second edition) *Evolutionary Psychiatry: A New Beginning*. London: Routledge.

Students During Covid-19 Lockdown. *European Child & Adolescent Psychiatry*, 17th February. https://link.springer.com/article/10.1007/s00787-021-01934-z [accessed 1st March, 2022]

Szasz T (1961) *The Myth of Mental Illness: Foundations of a Theory of Personal Conduct*. New York: Hoeber-Harper.

Szasz T (2007) *The Medicalization of Everyday Life: Selected Essays*. New York: Syracuse University Press.

Torrey, E and Miller, J (2002) *The Invisible Plague: The Rise of Mental Illness From 1750 to the Present*. New Brunswick, NJ, USA: Rutgers University Press.

Turner T and Machalek R (2018) *The New Evolutionary Sociology: Recent and Revitalized Theoretical and Methodological Approaches*. Abington-on-Thames: Routledge.

Whitaker R (2019) (revised edition) *Mad in America: Bad Science, Bad Medicine, and the Enduring Mistreatment of the Mentally Ill*. New York: Basic Books.Wilson EO (1975) *Sociobiology: The New Synthesis*. Cambridge, MA: Harvard University Press.

Wistrich H (2022) Can Women in Britain Ever Trust the Police Again? Here's What Must Happen First. *The Guardian*, 18th January. https://www.theguardian.com/commentisfree/2023/jan/18/women-britain-trust-met-police-david-carrick-sarah-everard [accessed 19th January, 2022]

World Health Organisation (2022a) Mental Health and COVID-19: Early Evidence of the Pandemic's Impact Scientific Brief, 2 March. file:///C:/Users/campb/Downloads/WHO-2019-nCoV-Sci-Brief-Mental-health-2022.1-eng.pdf [accessed 10th November, 2022]

World Health Organisation (2022b) *World Mental Health Report: Transforming Mental Health for All*. Geneva: World Health Organisation.

Yonker L, Boucau J, Regan J, Choudhary M, Burns M, Young N, Farkas E, Davis J, Moschovis P, Kinane T, Fasano A, Neilan A, Li J and Barczak A (2021) Virologic Features of Severe Acute Respiratory Syndrome Coronavirus 2 Infection in Children. *Journal of Infectious Diseases*, 224(11), pp.1821–1829.

4 Signs of Sanity

The world seems awash with human-made societal insanities. But the world is also brimming with signs of sanity. Kindness and cooperation, social solidarity, and coping and hoping, exist amongst the violence, inequality, selfishness, insecurity, and stupidity. Moreover, even in times of social crises when one or more of the societal insanities is running rampant (perhaps to the point of threatening all life on earth) kindness and cooperation, social solidarity, and coping and hoping, are also prevalent.

Kindness and Cooperation

Kindness is not strange. Cooperation not competitiveness is commonplace. That is kindness and cooperation are ordinary aspects of human performance. But what happens during extraordinary times? Are kindness and cooperation replaced by savagery, selfishness, strife, and survival of the fittest? Do plagues, pandemics, wars, and disasters bring out the better angels of human nature and nurture or release demons that are otherwise regulated by the superego and societal consciences and conventions? Human-to-human (and human-to-animal) kindness and cooperation and their opposites affect mental health. But is there a difference between these factors in normal and abnormal times?

Kindness covers personal performances and societal systems and structures that are either designed or fortuitously propagate kindliness. Personal kindly behaviours include acts of altruism, compassion, philanthropy, and magnanimity. Kindness, however, may be cognitive in the sense that an individual intends to be altruistic, compassionate, philanthropic, or magnanimous, and this is comprehended by the target of those intentions. That is, the act may not actually be enacted by the would-be giver, but the thought is appreciated by the would-be receiver. Kindliness may also involve emotions either as an element of an action or intended action, or as a stand-alone endeavour. That is, there is the realisation by the receiver that another person is 'feeling' kindly towards her/him. The expression 'I feel your pain' if received as a genuine emotional connection rather than a comical platitude is experienced as kindness.

Kindness will also include the operations of societal systems, structures, and institutions. For example, although some governments conduct cruelties

DOI: 10.4324/9781003223757-5

such as imprisoning political opponents and sanctioning extra-judicial killings, other regimes (along with non-government agencies) sanction kindnesses such as donating life-saving domestic and foreign aid in times of disaster. Not infrequently, governments perform paradoxically in an entangled enactment of intentional or unintentional benevolences and brutalities.

Claudia Hammond is a psychologist and broadcaster. One broadcast she presents is the BBC radio programme titled *All in the Mind* in which ideas and data about how humans think, feel and behave, are discussed with particular reference to mental health. Hammond suggests that there is evidence that humans are kinder than commonly supposed.

[T]here is a lot more kindness in the world already... Humanity outweighs inhumanity...

(Hammond, 2022, p.5)

Media news reporting and entertainment tend to focus on the sensational and unusual. An exaggerated impression of human capacity for cruelty and contrariness is the consequence of media concentrating on incidents of violence and narcissism. Malevolence, murder, immorality, and mayhem, make money. Everyday kindness and cooperation rarely hit the headlines, or if they do then they are presented as exceptional. Such overwhelming concentration on the bad poses a risk for psychological solidity, especially in those who already perceive themselves in a negative light. Sensing that the world is a wicked place and fellow humans are repeatedly callous and cussed is not likely to assuage existing feelings of apprehension and melancholy.

Hammond raises the issue of societal functionality in relation to kindness and cooperation. She argues that far from these qualities being the opposite of what is often contended as useful for personal success in the present-day global economic system or for the success of that system, they are beneficial. That is why they are commonplace. People need to support each other otherwise the system would fail. Equally, mutual interest means that systems need to collaborate as much if not more than they compete. Ironically, just as meanness and kindliness can co-exist, so can competitiveness and cooperativeness. Both individuals and organisations can and do accommodate these on the outwardly mutually exclusive facets.

Hammond reasons that Kindness is complicated. But that does not make kindness special. To repeat, all psychological, biological, and social ideas and actualities, are complex, and frequently contain elements of contradiction. Kindness, states Hammond, is also difficult to define and regularly misunderstood. Again, most popular, academic, and clinical concepts suffer from elucidatory imprecision and miscomprehension to a greater or lesser degree.

While kindness abounds, it still needs to be nurtured and propagated. Hammond calls for the fostering of a culture of kindness. The bidding by Hammond and her colleagues for more kindness and cultural changes towards kindliness is somewhat at odds with their claim that so much of it exists already. Perhaps the more suitable undertaking is to ensure that it is established as an essential norm for global society to be counted as sane.

Diminishing the coverage of unkindness in media might also have the effect of both raising the public's awareness that badness is not the norm and reducing the bad effect on emotional well-being of negative messaging on mental health. Hammond also takes to task some of the famous experiments by social scientists that have stressed how humans can be easily seduced into violent performances. These experiments include research by social psychologist Stanley Milgram (1974) in which participants were encouraged to give electric shocks to a person hidden from them but whose responses of agony they could hear. Milgram concluded that people obey out of fear of seeming to be uncooperative, especially if told to do something by a figure of authority. They will carry out these actions even when they are counter to their own values. What Hammond points out is that many of those commanded to shock others in Milgram's experiments refused to do so despite enormous pressure from the apparently respectable person in a white coat holding a clipboard ostensibly conducting research into a topic with no connection to obedience (let alone to be obediently unkind).

Campaigning for more kindness should include self-kindness. That is, kindness towards oneself is not, for Hammond, a discreditable indulgence, but an important precursor to the spreading of compassion amongst others. Hammond argues that mental health is bettered by self-kindness.

Human kindness and mental health have intricate and profound bonds. Kindness has a positive impact on the mental health of both the giver and receiver. Kindness can be an antidote to feelings of isolation, insecurity, self-doubt, and low self-worth, and can deepen friendships. Kindness helps make the world happier. Kindness is contagious (Mental Health Foundation, 2022b).

The effect of kindness on mental health goes further than those that reduce psychological suffering and increase the solidity of the psyche. There is neuroscientific evidence that kindly performances may make changes to the brain's physiology in a similar way to those that happen when levels of happiness and altruism are raised (Post, 2005; 2009). Kindness is not contrary to human nature (Hammond, 2022). There are specific parts of human brains, namely the mesolimbic pathway, that become active when stimulated by experiences of falling in love, eating chocolate, and by obtaining or performing kindnesses. So, the brain is ready to receive, react, and readjust to kindness. Moreover, more kindness is kind to the mind.

Kindness Test

Hammond is also involved with a major academic study on kindness conducted from 31 August 2021 until 4 October 2021. This study, named 'The Kindness Test' was based at the University of Sussex's Centre for Research on Kindness in the UK. It had the aim of investigating kindness and illuminating how kindness impacts of people and communities, and involved the completion of an online questionnaire by more than 60,000 adults from 144 countries (University of Sussex, 2023)

For the Kindness Test researchers, altruism and cooperation are linkable to kindness. As mentioned above, the issue of motivation means a more nuanced discernment is needed about how these three performances overlap. With some acts of altruism, there is a definite extrinsic cost that is realised by the giver. This could be physical and psychological energy, time, or money spent on charitable causes. The reward could be intrinsic, an example of which includes self-satisfaction with having helped. However, the intrinsic pay-off may not be realised at all. Some people may be 'hard-wired' to be kind, altruistic, and cooperative, and the meaning of their kindly, altruistic, and cooperative performances, may not reach a conscious level. They just do what comes 'naturally', whether this is primarily part of their nature or has become so because of the nurturing they have undergone. The same can be suggested about the cost of altruism, cooperativeness, and kindness. When there is the intention to benefit from kindly, altruistic, and cooperative performances, the expectation may be that this will be in the form of, for example, reciprocity, and reputational improvement.

Notwithstanding the nuanced approach to understanding the gradations and intricacies set-up by the Kindness Test researchers, they separate kindness into two seemingly opposing strands based on motivation. They label one of those strands 'altruistic kindness', which for them is when there is no obvious pay-off for the giver. The other strand they label 'strategic kindness', and as this descriptor implies, this a pay-off that is obvious for the giver.

Even more confusing is the Kindness Test researchers' imputation that kindness has neurological correlates, but that these are differ depending on whether the act is altruistic or strategic. This attempt to disentangle types of kindness by means measuring motivation seems to pander to simplification rather than the complexity inherent in all aspects of human performance, and which the Kindness Test researchers otherwise recognise. Moreover, by describing one type of kindness as 'altruistic' disregards how other theorists and empirical researchers regard them as either entwined or synonymous. Although there is an industrious academic and clinical study of motivation briming with assessment scales, and in part this is because finding out how people can be motivated is useful to industry, establishing exactly why people do or don't act in certain ways is extremely difficult. Motives vary over time, and fluctuate as behaviours, wants, needs, and external stimuli, change. Similar to other parts of human performance, motivation is not stable or unidirectional, it is a 'stream' of entangled cognitions and unconscious mechanisms, sind emotions. One dominant motive may be made up of a multitude of subsidiary motivations any one of which may become more imperative. Moreover, preceding and present biological, psychological, and societal factors will have and will continue to modify motives (Deckers, 2014).

More straightforwardly, the overlap of cooperation, altruism, and kindness is also acknowledged by the Kindness Test researchers when they petition that both are prerequisites for societal cohesion. Put simply, neither society nor humanity would exist if both had not embedded cooperation and kindness (whether kindness is denoted as altruistic or not) into their conjoint endeavours. Put practically, kindness is as kindness does, and the same can be said of cooperation. Motivation doesn't matter much if at all to the beggar given money or a meal by a stranger, nor if countries who own nuclear weapons sign a non-proliferation treaty and keep to their promises.

These researchers adopt a succinct definition of kindness as an act carried out to benefit others. Kindness is expressed in three ways for the team who conducted the Kindness Test research. These are as follows: (a) being kind; (b) receiving kindness; (c) observing kindness. All of these ways were more commonly reported by the study's female participants. Two results from the study have direct relevance to social crises and mental health. First, two-thirds of the participants reported that the COVID-19 pandemic has made people kinder. Participants who reported receiving, giving, or noticing, more acts of kindness also reported higher levels of emotional well-being.

Kindness seemed to select certain sites more than others in this study. Kindness was noted at home, in healthcare settings, the workplace, parks and other green areas, and shops. Kindness was noticed less on public transport, on the street, and when using the Internet. Kindness Test researchers suggest that family and community familiarity versus anonymity (especially when using social media) affect kindness. Apart from anonymity hindering kindness – and possibly an aperture through which unkindness can enter – so was a belief that a kindly act might be misinterpreted by the potential receiver. Therefore, the motivation of the receiver to accept, ignore, or refuse an act of kindness is also relevant.

Hammond comments that the essential and positive conclusion from the Kindness Test is that kindness is common. For her and the rest of the Kindness Test researchers, the data from the study indicating that kindness is unexceptional needs to be broadcast widely. Spreading the results of the Kindness Tests will, they argue, encourage yet more kindness to be generated in homes, communities, and workplaces.

Science writer specialising in neuroscience and psychology, Zara Abrams (2021), makes the case for kindness. There is much evidence, indicates Abrams, that being kind is not only morally worthwhile but there many benefits for the giver's physical and psychological health including boosting happiness and reducing blood pressure. Prosocial performance, whether towards family members, friends, strangers, or oneself, can be a spark for better well-being. The benefits occur whether an act of kindness is large or small in terms of effort, time, and money. Regarding small kindnesses, Abrams provides examples of holding the door open for a stranger, bringing coffee to a colleague, and petting an animal (there is more about kindness to animals below). Her example of large kindness is helping a friend to move house. Observing or recalling the delivery of kindness is also a catalyst for physical and psychological enhancement. Improvements in physical health can facilitate psychological solidity. Therefore, any indication that kindness is related to better mental health is important to note. One study mentioned by Abrams examined the impact of kindness on genes (Nelson-Coffey *et al.*, 2017). The conclusion of the study is that there is a causal effect of prosocial performance on the regulation of leukocyte genes. That is, being kind has a positive effect the immunological system.

Not all acts of kindness, however, are equal argues Abrams. Taking the example of generosity, she suggests that giving directly rather than indirectly is more beneficial for the giver. That is, donating face-to-face to a charity collector or handing cash to someone *impecunious state sparks more benefits than donating online. This is because the evidence, submits Abrams, that direct generosity personalises the act and increases social connectedness. It provides immediate emotional rewards for the giver and may also do so for the receiver. Freely chosen generosity is also more beneficial than when this occurs because of peer or wider societal pressure. What is even less beneficial is if a gift is not only given because it is required or demanded. When force is involved, it is questionable whether the act can be categorised as kind.*

More than merely making the case for kindness, Abrams campaigns for it to spread. An example of her activism is her encouragement for people to engage with a challenge hosted by the Born This Way Foundation for young people to indulge in more kindness performances from 1 September to 21 September 2021. The purpose of this campaign was to 'foster mental wellness' by helping to build kinder and more cooperative communities (Born This Way Foundation, 2023). Individuals, schools, non-profit organisations, and corporations were invited to 'pledge' to be kinder by signing-up through social media using the hashtag #BeKind21. They were also asked share their experiences of being kind. Over 6.8 million participants pledged to conduct 143 million acts of kindness.

Human history, according to psychologist Steven Pinker (2011) and historian Rutger Bregman (2020) kindness and cooperativeness are notable for a decreasing commitment to violence and solitariness. Humans can be bad but are more frequently good.

Kindness to Animals

What about human kindness towards and cooperation with other life forms? Does the keeping by humans of animals as surrogate family members and friends outweigh the billions of animals that have been slaughtered for human food and hunted for human pleasure each year, the colossal number kept in inhuman conditions on farms and in markets, and used as a means of transporting goods and people, and in previous epochs recruited in their millions to 'cooperate' with humans to kill other humans? Paradoxically, the ill-treatment and forced assistance that is inflicted on animals for the benefit of humanity have also caused catastrophe. Human health and animal husbandry are interlinked. It is probable that COVID-19 is a zoonotic disease, but if not, then there are plenty of other candidates for this category of animal-to-human contagion. The Centers for Disease Control and Prevention (2022) lists about 100 diseases that spread from animals and/or from humans to animals. These include bubonic plague, tuberculosis, bovine spongiform encephalopathy ('Mad Cow Disease'), *E. coli* (*Escherichia coli*), various Herpes infections, Lyme disease, monkeypox, rabies, swine influenza, salmonella, scabby mouth, and ticks.

Hence, kinder animal husbandry and human health are interlinked. Zoonotic diseases demonstrate well that connection. Labour studies scholar Kendra Coulter (2020) argues that the COVID-19 pandemic shows that humans must 'get serious' about the well-being of animals. Coulter observes that COVID-19 has raised many questions about global economics and politics. It is not only widespread disease that raises such questions but all social crises. However, seldom has any previous social crisis focused world attention on how animals are reared. The climate emergency broaches this issue because the widescale farming of animals for human consumption is extremely detrimental to ecological systems. The way humans manage fellow creatures has long been an ethical concern for animal welfare groups, veterinary professionals, and some governments.

At this point, I will make full disclosure regarding my ethical stance towards animals. I have been a vegetarian since September 1986. A pub meal of 'chicken-in-the-basket' was my last intake of meat (or fish), at least knowingly so. For the last few years my diet has been mostly vegan. I also been a trustee for the UK Vegetarian Society. Although there are benefits to the health of both humans and other animals and for the health of the planet, my reason for not eating animals is ethical. Sentient beings of any sort should not, in my view, suffer unnecessarily and while there are non-sentient sources of nutrition I chose not to add to the already high levels of suffering from human exploitation of animals. But I am not a sentimentalist about animals. Predator animals can be merciless to their prey, and even non-carnivorous varieties may conduct cruelties on weaker or non-related members of their and other species. Nor do I indulge in anthropomorphism. Animals may be sentient, but they are not humans.

The reader therefore should take account of my stance regarding animals and inspect what follows with that in mind. That said, my main concern in this book is not to campaign for vegetarianism or veganism other than when there is evidence that faulty animal husbandry is relatable to social crises and therefore mental health – which it is.

Coulter points out that human families, communities, and economic systems include animals. It can be argued that humans and animals are both in conflict in relation to the environment. But is humanity that is responsible for its own ecological misdemeanours and most of those caused by other creatures? Humans deliberately exploit animals on a massive scale. Animals only exploit humans in any deliberate sense when they are provided with food, shelter, and protection. But rarely are those benefits supplied unconditionally. Apart from being an unwitting source of contagion and conflict, animals unwittingly provide humans with nutritional sustenance, company for lonely people, assist in the socialisation of children, supply a means of transport, and a variety of forms of sport and entertainment.

There is also a contradiction in the conditional connection humans have with animals. While one animal species or a select few from a species, savours human attention, others are exploited, neglected, or slaughtered in their billions by humans. One notable contradiction involves the ownership of pets. Pet owners in the main feed their animals with the remains of other animals. Most pet food is made-up of either wet or dry mashed animal by-products bulked with vegetables and cereals. Apart from the ethical enigma of feeding animals to animals, the practice has caused contagion and aggravated the climate emergency.

The global environmental 'paw print' of pet food has been assessed as huge. More than half of global human households own a companion animal, mostly a cat of dog. A study of dry pet-food alone concluded that agricultural land roughly twice the size of the UK is used annually to make dry food for cats and dogs. Annual greenhouse gas emissions were found to be equivalent to total emissions from countries such as Mozambique or the Philippines (Alexander *et al.*, 2020).

The UK charity the Mental Health Foundation (2022a) lists the psychological pay-off for people for their pets. These include companionship and comforting; increased exercise from walking with a dog, which can also engender contact with likeminded people; a; reduction in anxiety, and an increase in self-confidence and motivation; the perception of unconditional affection; providing purposeful routine to daily activities, and a sense achievement and responsibility. What the Mental Health Foundation also point out is that pets can help with specific types of psychological states. Pets can encourage people diagnosed with Attention Deficit and Hyperactivity Disorder to maintain a structure to their day, and/or release excessive energy. The feeling that a pet is listening and loving without prerequisites or judgements may assist people diagnosed with autism to be more trustful, calm, and confident, as well as reduce fear of tactility.

Therefore, there are costs and benefits to human and animal interactions for both. But Coulter surmises that the cost of animal suffering is present and prospective human suffering. Humans being kindlier to animals is crucial, she argues, for the future of humanity. Coulter affirms that she is not campaigning on behalf of vegans and against omnivores, but for the future of life on Earth. But in effect, her case is one supporting veganism (not vegetarianism if dairy products or still consumed) because humans eating far fewer animals, or none, would have dramatically reduced the risk from the dangers she identifies.

It is for Coulter the consumption of animals, and how they are fed, farmed, and vended, that has intensified the danger of further pandemics. Millions of viruses inhabit animals. When humans come into contact with animals they are also in contact with these viruses, some of which are very dangerous to human health and for which there are no vaccines to prevent disease or cures if contracted. This is on top of the serious situation with antibiotic resistance whereby the overuse of these drugs in animals has led to a growing threat to humans who are suffering from bacterial infections, possibly as a result of a preceding viral illness that may have been contracted from animals.

Coulter has three recommendations to deal with human cataclysmic capitalisation of their fellow creatures. First, the cross-border trade in millions of exotic animals such as monkeys, turtles, snakes, should be stopped. Second, the industrialisation and corporatisation of animal husbandry, slaughtering, and marketing, need to be curtailed, and encouragement given to sustainable agriculture, plant-based foods and drinks, and lab-grown meat and milk. Third, the idea of 'one health' whereby human, animal and environmental health are recognised as inextricably linked needs to be central to personal lifestyle choices and adopted by policymakers. It is the responsibility of national governments and international agencies dealing with the welfare of humans, animals, and the environment to rectify this social crisis.

Coulter concludes her argument that humans must get serious about the well-being of animals with this plea:

> The animals deserve better, and so does our species. A simple return to the status quo is not only unjust, it is dangerous.
>
> (Coulter, 2020)

If only the selfish reason of humanity's survival, humans need to be kind to animals. But kindness to animals is also an indication that human society is becoming more morally civilised.

Disasters and Kindness

Commenting on how people behave during crises, science journalist Laura Spinney (2017) suggests that most people when the opportunity arises, act altruistically. Spinney queries whether apparent selflessness is, paradoxically, clandestine selfishness. But even if this is so it doesn't negate the positive effects of self-interest and contributes to 'collective resilience'. Most health workers during the Spanish flu stayed to care for their patients despite the risk to them of catching the disease, and when they became ill lay people took over.

Cooperation and discord can coexist. The medieval plagues and 17th Great Plague of London sowed widespread death and destruction. Historian Paul Slack (1988), however, this devastating disease also elicited positive social responses. One prime example of the positivity that plague propagated was to bring to the forefront a responsibility national and local authorities had to diminish the effects of the disease on their populations to defend them from future outbreaks. For Slack, the techniques used at the time of the plague epidemics to control its spread or prevent it occurring shaped subsequent concepts and practices of public health:

> Plague victims were isolated and their contacts traced and incarcerated. There were restrictions on movement, bills of health, quarantine regulations for travelers and shipping. Bedding and houses were fumigated.
>
> (Slack, 1988, p.433)

Slack also notes that instilling, monitoring, and enforcing these mechanisms needed a sizable growth of local and State administrative systems and increased the number and power of officials. These measures were highly controversial at the time, although eventually followed to a greater or lesser extent by most people. However, restrictions on individual liberty and on the running of businesses by what Slack denotes as the 'medical police' were resisted by a sizeable minority of the affected populations. Others had taken their personal health measure by fleeing the infected area, and by doing so possibly infecting those they had contact with on route and at their destination.

What can also co-exist is cruelty and compassion. Slack comments that what at first consideration seems ruthless measure of self-protection and the protection of close relatives was the refusal to help friends, neighbours, and distant members of the family, and the turning out into the streets anyone in the household who has become noticeably infected. But Slack points out that this was an understandable measure in the circumstances. Moreover, what also occurred was the exact opposite of sensible personal-preserving precautions. Rather than shunning those outside the household, help was commonly offered to friends, neighbours, and distant relatives. Although the formation of 'medical policing' meant more surveillance and regulation of the public, it was indicative of how systems and structures of governance has been maintained even when so many people, including operatives of those systems and structures, were dying or dead and many social institutions had shut down.

But callousness, as Slack comments, may also have been disguised as kindness. He refers to how double standards operated in Italian towns. The poor were forcibly removed from their homes and placed in special 'plague hospitals', the lazarettos. They therefore were separated from the rats and fleas carrying the disease, their bedding burned, and their homes fumigated as best as was possible without modern disinfectants. This may on the surface appear to be a magnanimous measure. But these lazarettos, however, were overcrowded and disease-spreading hotspots. Rich people were allowed to stay in their own homes along with their servants, although this did mean they continued to be in contact with the domestic rats with their fleas, and materials, that the poor were now avoiding.

The conclusion Slack comes to regarding how people and the authorities responded to the plague is that hard choices had to be made. He emphasises this point by giving the example of the dilemma faced by the government from 1720 to 1722 when plague from Marseilles threatened. The government decided that if the plague did arrive, then those who were infected would be confined in pesthouses, and troops would be stationed around London with orders to shoot anyone who attempted to leave the city so that the rest of the country would be protected.

Medieval historian Samuel Cohn's (2018) study of 'hate and compassion' during major disease outbreaks such as the plague, the Great Influenza of 1918–1919, and AIDS leads him to the opposite conclusion to what he suggests is the usual picture painted about personal and societal performances. For Cohn what is commonly found is not selfishness and social disintegration but self-sacrifice and social integration, and these positive attributes are found across social classes, and race, ethnic, and religious groupings. Throughout history disease outbreaks have, argues Cohn, brought people together through, for example, acts of compassion and volunteerism. Societal cohesiveness benefits from, for example, improved medical knowledge, building better housing, safer water supplies, improving waste disposal, and by showing up the credibility of public health as a general approach to disease prevention and management.

Maia Szalavitz (2012) is a neuroscience journalist obsessed with addiction, love, evidence-based living, empathy and pretty much everything related to the brain and behaviour. She argues that it is natural for humans in times of calamity to become more kind and more cooperative. Survival is core to human nature (and all other forms of life). Kindness and cooperativeness increase the chances of individuals and their genetic relations of coping with disasters. For Szalavitz there is a popular misconception that disasters arouse frenzied selfishness and brutal survival-of-the-fittest competitiveness. What is more common is altruism, states Szalavitz. She cites situations of natural calamities such as the 2012 tropical storm-force 'Hurricane Sandy' that affected countries from the Caribbean to Canada, killing hundreds of people and causing US$ billions worth of damage. Reports of looting and other crimes of opportunity were apparently minimal whereas accounts of people helping each other abounded. This help included people checking on vulnerable neighbours, sharing food and providing shelter, and offering general support. Szalavitz also mentions the years of the Blitz when London was bombed relentlessly during the Second World War, and aeroplanes hit and brought down the Twin Towers in New York on 11 September 2001. On both occasions, suggests Szalavitz, compassion and solidarity were apparent during the aftermath, and she adds that this has been the case following most major earthquakes or tsunamis wherever in the world they have occurred.

Historian Rutger Bregman (2020) notes that during **the blitz years** that devastated cities such as London, Coventry, Liverpool, and Southampton, there was undoubtedly a high level of emotional distress caused by the high level of human causalities and destruction of property, but there was no mass despondency nor were there mass admissions into psychiatric institutions. Bregman (2020) argues that the mental health of the populations living in Blitzed cities improved, and there was a reduction in alcoholism. Far from a breaking down of morale as had been the goal of the Nazi regime, more evident during the blitz were displays of courageousness, humour, and kindness. What manifested was shared support, not selfish survivalism.

Bregman is pointing to the paradoxes of warfare. The occurrence of humans killing humans occurs alongside comradeship and camaraderie. Soldiers and civilians on the respective sides of armed conflicts seek solidarity. For Bregman, when a social crisis occurs humans reveal the better angels of their nature. There are, of course, exceptions and these are frequently over-emphasised because of media coverage. Disasters in the main do not engender mass hysteria or rampant crime. Most people even when faced with the effects and after-effects of catastrophe, argues Bregman, stay calm. Many will take actions to help both themselves and others cope. For Bregman, it is because humans are social animals that they continue to crave the company of other humans despite and because of catastrophe.

Hurricane Katrina devastated the USA city of New Orleans and surrounding areas in August 2005. The storm and resultant floods led to the death of more than 1,300 people died as a direct result of the storm and subsequent floods, and hundreds of thousands were displaced. Rumours and media reports spread about looting, hijacking, and rioting, some of which were to be verified as having happened. But what did not get as much attention, at least in the early stages of the aftermath, were the far more common instances of altruism, cooperativeness, and camaraderie within the affected communities and between survivors and the emergency services personnel. Social solidarity surfaced rather than savagery and selfishness. According to a public health report published by epidemiologist Binu Jacob and her colleagues in which the evidence about human performance during disasters is examined, common assumptions about how people behave are erroneous (Jacob *et al.*, 2008). Focusing on Hurricane Katrina, Binu Jacob and her colleagues argue that misconceptions about the reactions of individuals and communities when caught in disasters prevail despite considerable empirical evidence to the contrary. Acts of misconduct and Mayhem are submerged under waves of compassion and generosity. This is so no matter whether the disaster is 'natural' or human-made. The authors of the report challenge ten 'myths'.

The first myth challenged in this report is that international medical help is urgently needed. This may be necessary for specialist treatments but otherwise the local lay population and medical personnel from the surrounding areas usually manage to deal with immediate medical requirements. Another myth debunked is that any kind of international assistance and lots of it is needed as soon as possible. This is not the case as too much to quickly adds to the chaos that is likely when disasters happen. Outside support may be welcome but only after an assessment has been made about need by those affected and their local and national authorities. What is also challenged in the report is the notion that deadly diseases are inevitable in the aftermath of disasters. There is increased risk if dead bodies are left to rot, sanitation systems are broken, water supplies are inadequate or contaminated, and overcrowding occurs amongst displaced populations. But threats to health post-disaster can be lessened if public health measures are already at hand especially within or near areas known prone to catastrophe, and if emergency services are adequately staffed and equipped and ready to respond.

In relation to kindness and cooperation, Jacob and her co-researchers insist that disasters do not in the main bring out the worst in people. They like others collating robust evidence rather than assenting to misleading mythology, counsel that anti-social acts such as looting and rioting is heavily outweighed by a multitude of prosocial performances. Examples of the latter include community leaders promoting a positive attitude regarding the potential to cope and regaining hope, and actual resilience amongst survivors. Further performances of pro-sociability noted by Jacob *et al.* are multiple displays of generosity. Generosity in disasters situations can range from simple acts of sharing food and water, providing clothing and blankets. Greater degrees of generosity may arise from those whose homes have not been destroyed by a disaster by offering accommodation and emotional comfort to people who have been made homeless and may have also lost loved ones as a result of a hurricane or missile.

Jacob and her co-researchers argue that despite risk of injury or death humans are not necessarily motivated to seek personal safety. The drive to seek safety may be negated by the drive to seek the familiar in terms of locality and people. This contrary reaction can explain why emergency service personnel and officials have difficultly removing people from their disaster-hit surroundings, and if removal is insisted on by the authorities there is equal insistence by survivors that they should be accompanied by family and/or friendship groups. This reaction by survivors is yet another indication of how people are wanting to operate collectively, and in so doing supply and receive support. Mutuality and selflessness are apparent rather than discord and selfishness.

On the theme of physical danger being generally far less stressful than separation from familiar people and surroundings, Jacob and her colleagues refer to the reactions of children in London who were living with the daily danger of being hurt or killed due to the blitzkrieg bombing 1940–1941.

[C]hildren showed few signs of distress, even if exposed to scenes of death and violence, if they were with a parent or with schoolmates and teachers; it was only if they were separated from parents or other attachment figures under these conditions that serious psychological disturbances occurred.

(Jacob *et al.*, 2008, p.564)

Signs of (emotional) distress also surfaced amongst people who were forced to relocate because their homes had not been destroyed but damaged. The damage was sufficient for the authorities to consider it unsafe to stay in these homes. But for the occupiers of these homes, the risk was worth taking rather than risks posed through resettlement. People who were evacuated when Hurricane Katrina hit showed in the following months increased levels of moderate and severe symptoms of PTSD.

For Jacob and her co-researchers in times of disaster, there are profound adverse physical and psychological consequences from separation from or the loss of people and surroundings with whom there are strong emotional and environmental bonds. These researchers emphasise that maintaining social attachments is essential for preserving psychological and physical well-being when affected by disaster. Interpersonal and community connections and connections to a locale are essential for preserving psychological and physical well-being in non-disaster times. But that this relationship should be so in times of disaster is not only significant but surprising.

Psychologist Lacy Margana and her colleagues (Margana *et al.*, 2019) point out that there is much evidence that prosocial performance in males makes them more attractive to females as potential mates. Altruism, in particular, seems to be a sexual signal. Margana and her colleagues consider heroism as an element of prosocial performance. What they explore is the synergic value of heroism and altruism in mate selection. These researchers conclude men who display both altruism and heroism do increase their desirability rating amongst potential female mates. They add, however, that altruistic and heroic men increase their chances further if they are regarded also as physically attractive by females. In a further nuance to their findings, Margana and her colleagues suggest that these attributes in men are given more value by females seeking long-term rather than short-term relationships. It is unclear exactly what differences in desirability occur in different levels of single or synergetic elements of prosocial performance. For example, would an exceptionally high level of heroics override the absence of altruism when females select a mate? There is the assumption in such research that prosocial performance can be disaggregated into discrete components. While altruism can be separated from heroism, the reverse is problematic. As with altruism (and every other aspect of human performance) motivation and context matter when it comes to heroism. There is a deep difference, for example, between a heroic emotional and cognitive reformation to overcoming a phobia and the heroic act of saving a wounded comrade on the battlefield. Moreover, many people perform everyday heroics in managing gruelling circumstances such as trying to find food for the family when living in dire destitution or saving an animal from drowning in a raging torrent. These days some of these everyday heroics could be captured on camera and subsequently shown to millions via an internet video site or shared on social media. But most of these 'mini social crises' will be accomplished anonymously. The psychological payoff heroics may also differ depending on the level of recognition. If unobserved a heroic performance may still serve as a stimulus for self-satisfaction. If widely observed, then the psychological payoff may be magnified or offset by fame and/or financial benefits.

Heroic Kindness

Rather than continuing to fixate on everyday minor misfortunes, there is a raising of consciousness and conscientiousness about the misfortune of others when disasters occur. People seem to soon realise the seriousness of a situation in times of catastrophe when their love-ones, neighbours, pets, and even strangers are in danger of injury or death. During disasters and in their aftermath, there are as many if not more heroic deeds as there are felonious feats. At times standard social restrictions and superficial interpersonal niceties are superseded by what seems like superhuman struggles to save lives. However, what soon becomes regularised and normalised are small altruisms, kindnesses, and cooperations, rather than outstandingly brave performances. But heroics, especially when they gain media attention, are, of course, appreciated by those who have been rescued from raging rivers or burning buildings. Heroics also serve to enhance community cohesion and provide an antidote to cynical views of humanity.

Political, environmental, and feminist activist and historian, Rebecca Solnit, argues that disasters bring forth a surge in altruism. In her book titled *A Paradise Built in Hell: The Extraordinary Communities That Arise in Disaster* (2008) Solnit examines different disasters and concludes that these events bring out the best in humanity. Solnit's examples also include Hurricane Katrina and the London Blitz, as well as the Chornobyl nuclear catastrophe. People and communities pull together and engage in a common cause has been observed during the COVID-19 pandemic and the war in Ukraine, and these two social crises have also demonstrated how nations pull together with other nations. But Solnit argues, the reaction of governments to the disasters she cites may well have hindered the more immediate and apposite responses of people directly involved. For Solnit, top-down measures may inhibit the extraordinary efforts of communities.

Notwithstanding outstanding obstacles such as governmental counterproductive policies, personal agency comes into play with a display of extraordinary performance. These individuals are the ones identified as heroes for their bravery, improvisation, and immediacy. They are the people who either nature or nurture has endowed with the perceptual promptness, physical prowess, and unfettered self-confidence to act and face danger when others in are danger. The appropriate social milieu is necessary, however, for heroics to be judged as such. Extant and/or post-event audiences and whoever has been saved from injury or death must interpret the intervention as valiant and not self-indulgent or senseless, and the environmental conditions must be aligned in such a way to allow derring-do opportunities.

The distribution of kindness and cooperation is uneven. Kindness and cooperation will be displaced by ingroup and outgroup divisions, geographical and temporal distances, and historical disagreements, between different countries and cultures. (Hammond, 2022). But kindness and cooperation can also transcend these patterns when disaster strikes. For example, politicians might make the wrong decision when faced with social crises, but they can also act heroically by overcoming long-term bitterness embedded in their country's culture.

The debacle of the economy of Greece during the first two decades of the 21st century, the requirement for strict fiscal controls as a condition for a series of billions of euros in loans made by the European Union (mainly German banks) and the International Monetary Fund, resulted in mass unemployment, a huge rise in poverty, and large-scale social unrest and the further widening of political divisions and disarray. Despite this drastic situation for Greece, writer of historical books James Heneage comments on how community still mattered:

> The Greeks endured not just because they had no choice but because they still had something others had lost: community. Many young people moved back to their villages. Churches opened their doors … [T]he medical profession opened 'solidarity clinics' across the country, run by volunteer doctors assisted by local citizens.
>
> (Heneage, 2022, p.228)

At another time, old rivalries that has involved wars and territorial disputes over millennia between Turks (Ottomans) and Greeks, and conflict between these two NATO allies continues today (Erdem, 2022). But this discord has been on occasions put aside. Writer of historical books James Heneage notes that Greeks and Turks are supposed to be enemies, but as Athens was gripped by famine in early years of the Second World War, Turkish ships supplied the city with grain Turkey. The German occupiers had stripped Greece of much of the populations basic means of survival including raw industrial materials and food to equip and feed its troops fighting elsewhere in Europe. The exact number of deaths from starvation (as well as disease due to vulnerability caused by malnutrition, polluted or absent water, and the lack of shelter, clothes, and heating) is not known. Heneage suggests it could have been 200,000 during the winter of 1941–1942. The exact number of Greeks saved by Turkish kindness is also not known. But one of their ships saved one thousand starving and traumatised Greek children by backing them to safety in Turkey.

Reciprocal kindness was shown when in 1999 an earthquake struck the Turkish town of Izmit and it also affected Istanbul. It killed more than 17,000 people. Greece was the first country to offer and then send emergency aid and rescue workers. A month later Athens had its own earthquake and Turkey responded in a similar humanitarian fashion to that of Greece (Erdem, 2022).

In 2023, The Greeks once more were one of the first if not the first to offer help their Turkish neighbours when powerful earthquakes and then a series of aftershocks hit the south of Turkey as well as the north of Syria. Thousands of people died in this disaster and there was widespread destruction to buildings and infrastructure. The Prime Minister of Greece, Kyriakos Mitsotakis, is reported to have telephoned the Turkish President Recep Tayyip Erdoğan offering condolences and immediate assistance in the form of rescuers and supplies when the first earthquake struck. This is despite a resurgence of tensions between the two countries and the severing of diplomatic communications the previous year (Al Jazeera, 2023).

The COVID-19 pandemic brought to the forefront of the media and public's attention the occurrence of heroism. Many of those considered heroes remained anonymous while others became famous. In countries such as the UK, front-line workers and emergency personnel were on mass construed as heroic for performing under the demanding and dangerous circumstances of a deadly disease spreading rapidly across the world. Doctors, nurses, ambulance operatives, and social care staff, were faced with the number of debilitated and dying people rising exponentially as the disease was, at least in the early months, out of the control of the authorities or was denied as a real risk to health by some of those in authority. The hero ascription was applied to more and more groups of workers as the pandemic continued and worsened. Food delivery drivers, retailers working in premises that were allowed to stay open or re-opened, and public transport staff managing the few buses and trains permitted to operate, were lauded for their exceptional community spirit.

Individuals who had performed exceptional personal feats also become household names. One of those is Thomas Moore or 'Captain Tom' as he became known to the British public. Thomas Moore was born in April 1920. He was conscripted into the British army in June 1940, and commissioned as an officer a year later. He served most of the years of the Second World War in India and Burma. In 1944 he was promoted to the rank of Captain (Moore, 2020).

Just before COVID-19 arrived and spread in the UK, Captain Tom had been receiving care from a nurse after he had fractured his hip. The nurse had advised him to 'keep mobile', and this he did by doing laps around his garden using a 'walker'. Eventually, he came up with the idea of walking to gain funds for the NHS. The idea came to him just as the first lockdown in the UK had started, March 2020. He intended only to do 100 laps to raise £1,000 (about US$1,223). The 100 lap target was significant for Captain Tom. He was 100-years-of-age the following month. He succeeded in accomplishing the 100 laps, but the money that was donated after the media took up his story far exceeded his target of £1,000. Three years after Captain Sir Tom started to do laps around his garden, the charitable foundation set-up in his name had received in donations nearly £40 million (Captain Tom Foundation, 2023). Captain Tom became Captain Sir Tom when he was knighted by

Queen Elizabeth II in July 2020. Captain Sir Tom died in February 2021. His legacy is one of popular hero and substantial charity fund raiser. The Captain Tom Foundation's website contains the following missive in which heroism is connected to hopefulness:

> Inspiring Hope Where it is Needed Most: Stories are what inspire us, stories of the ordinary turned extraordinary – the heroes of our everyday.
>
> (Captain Tom Foundation, 2023)

The hope mentioned here refers to Captain Sir Tom and the Foundation's support for the NHS, combatting of loneliness, and championing education, equality, and ageism. What is also hoped is that such stories will inspire psychological solidity.

However, there were multitudes of unsung heroes. One of these otherwise anonymous heroes is, however, 'sung' as a hero by the United Nations Children's Fund.[1] Judith Candiru is a Ugandan nurse. Nurse Candiru's usual day begins early when she collects water from a borehole, carries 20 litres balanced on her head back home, makes breakfast for her three children, and then heads off to work before heading off to work. Part of her nursing responsibilities in the Yumbe District of northern Uganda is carried out in the local clinics, the rest on visiting those patients who can't travel in their homes. She also attends local facilities such as markets and trading centres. Her mode of transport is a motorcycle, or she walks. In these locales, she uses a megaphone to deliver advice about how to gain and maintain good health and when to seek medical advice (United Nations Children's Fund, 2022a).

Unfortunately, Candiru contracted COVID-19. More unfortunately she, along with her family, was stigmatised and shunned by the very community she served. That time she describes as the 'saddest moment' of her career. But once she had recovered from the disease, she went back to serving her community throughout the COVID-19 pandemic. Her megaphonic message at this stage was one of encouraging people to get vaccinated (United Nations Children's Fund, 2022b).

The website page that records Candiru's story and those of similar 'unsung pandemic heroes' from around the world points to what may be the motivation to conduct extraordinary feats:

> For some it's a sense of duty. For others it's an obligation. And then there are those for which it's a necessity…. [E]xtraordinary women and men have risen to the occasion to serve their communities. Their names aren't necessarily recognizable. But the actions of these heroes have without a shadow of a doubt made our world a safer, better place.
>
> (United Nations Children's Fund, 2022b)

Although the above quotation designates these heroes as 'extraordinary, their extraordinariness only became reified in trying circumstances. Up until then, they were ordinary in the sense that their heroics had not been noted let alone sung. There remain countless people who do the extraordinary as part of their ordinary routines. Candiru is a case in point. Everyday she is fetching water, caring for her children, working in a responsible position, and probably also handling dozens of what for her are ordinary – and necessary – other tasks without the intrusion of a deadly disease. The intrusion of COVID-19 accentuated rather than invent heroism.

There is an equivalent of this contagion accentuated heroism during conflicts. There is a vibrant documentation of heroism that occurred in the two world wars. Many soldiers and civilians have been recognised and awarded for their bravery. The same is likely to happen in the Ukraine war. Captain Tom is a different story because he became a hero not during armed conflict exemplified by guns and bombs but when a virus became weaponised.

But most civilians and soldiers in zones of conflict, if not injured, starving, or killed, just get on with living as best as they can or fighting as they have been trained. For those observing from the outside (and these days most of the rest the world's population can do that through the widescale and immediate reporting of events in the media), to live in such situations demands astonishing fortitude. It also demands cooperation and kindness. Correctly, there is much made of the psychological suffering caused by conflict. There is inevitably a negative effect on the emotional stability of civilians and soldiers in zones of conflict, some of which will be severe and may not be appreciated as such at the time if ever. But most people if not seriously mentally debilitated will continue to cope.

The personal and societal payoffs from heroism are striking. The mental health of the hero may be improved, and social stability secured. The publicising of heroism can diminish emotional damage, motivate creativity, promote personal growth, and inspire community and wider societal identification and integration (Scott and Goethals, 2010). However, the publicising of heroics may serve the powerful by diverting the attention of the public from entrenched social problems. Further advantage for the powerful can be gained if acts of heroism are construed as the outcome or supportive of extant political and economic policies. In this light, it could be that the laudable and sincere heroism of Captain Tom became either by default or design presented to the British public by the State as implicitly integral to the drive for community adherence to the government's public health measures directed at dealing with the COVID-19 pandemic. These measures included the governmental attempting to generate *esprit de corps* amongst the population and to recognise both the centrality of the NHS and the pressures it was under coping with the influx of COVID-19 patients. When Captain Tom died (from the complications of COVID-19), Prime Minister Boris Johnson broadcast a tribute to him. In the tribute, Johnson states that Captain Tom was:

[A] hero in the truest sense of the word. In dark days of the Second World War he fought for freedom, and in the face of this country's deepest post-war crisis he united us all, he cheered us all up, and he embodied the triumph of the human spirit.

(Johnson, 2021)

Johnson also mentions in the tribute how Captain Tom's charitable contribution has assisted the efforts of NHS staff to continue to protect the public during the pandemic, and how he was not only a national inspiration by a 'beacon of hope' for the world.

Captain Tom had the cooperation of the British media and public when raising funds for charity during COVID-19. After he died the foundation set-up in his name continued to benefit from his fortitude. Captain Tom also wrote an autobiography (Moore, 2020) and a book in which he lists his life's lessons (Moore, 2021). These include be comfortable with who you are; keep smiling through the tough times; have an open mind; live life purposefully; try to understand the other's person's perspective; and eat porridge. However, his book is titled *Captain Tom's Life Lessons: Above All Be Kind*.

The designation of hero will depend on perception. Depending on which side in a war has the most effective propaganda, heroes will proliferate on the basis of not only bravery but good versus evil, and the immensity of the odds against surviving a valiant act. It will also depend of who ultimately wins the war. There are few Nazi heroes except amongst present-day far right groups. The ongoing (at the time of writing) Russian invasion of Ukraine has thrown up heroes on both sides. The 'Official Website of Ukraine' (2023) lists its 'defenders of freedom', while President Putin posits that the Russian Troops taking part in the war who are 'defending the fatherland' heroically (Putin, 2023).

Besides heroics, whether asserted or authentic, the war in Ukraine has undoubtedly dispensed horrors. The activist organisation 'Global Citizen', however, has highlighted the kindness of strangers. In an article written by content coordinator Nora Holz and editor Tess Lowery at Global Citizen website are acts of kindness that Global Citizen regards as showing shared human solidarity and compassion soon after Russia invaded Ukraine. These acts in the month following after Russia invaded Ukraine include Polish citizens setting up mobile kitchens at the border to feed the millions of fleeing refugees and leaving prams for those with babies, people offering accommodation to Ukrainian families displaced from their own homes, and hundreds of thousands of people in cities across the world protesting against the violence (Holz and Lowery, 2022).

Historian and political philosopher Hannah Arendt used the phrase 'the banality of evil' to describe how unexceptional humans can perform extraordinarily brutalities. The focus for her thesis is one of the main arrangers of the holocaust, Adolf Eichmann. An opposing thesis is suggested by PhD psychology student Zeno Franco and psychologist Philip Zimbardo. They use the descriptor 'the banality of heroism' to argue that although circumstances can instil inaction or participation in evil acts, they can also encourage bravery (Franco and Zimbardo, 2016). Moreover, Franco and Zimbardo suggest most people are capable of everyday heroism. Poignantly, Zimbardo is famous for 'Stanford Prison Experiment' in which ordinary young men were randomly assigned roles as 'prisoners' or 'guards' in a simulated prison. Those assigned the role of guard soon began using increasingly degrading forms of punishment against the prisoners. Those assigned the role of prisoner soon became passive. The conclusion reached by Zimbardo and his fellow researchers from that study was that under certain ordinary people can commit acts that would otherwise be unthinkable (Zimbardo *et al.*, 1973).

Social Solidarity

There are two types of solidarity, personal and social. Political theorist Lawrence Wilde provides a definition of personal solidarity:

> [A] feeling of sympathy shared by subjects within and between groups, impelling supportive action and pursuing social inclusion.
>
> (Wilde, 2013, p.1)

Social solidarity is the net effect of these personal contributions as well as the overarching input from the 'sum of society' being greater than the sum of its parts. Wilde examines how personal and social solidarity are contained within a globalised societal system. For him, globalisation is the process of increasing interconnectedness between social systems that are connected to particular cultures and countries. Wilde notes, however, it is the development of a worldwide interconnected economy, especially through the influences of transnational corporations and the World trade organisation, World Bank, and the International Monetary Fund, that dominates the values and norms inherent in globalisation. For Wilde, this lopsided dominance that favours big business and international trading standards at the expense of small business, local groups, and individuals, has manufactured what he terms a 'democratic deficit'.

One of the founders of sociology as an academic discipline, Emile Durkheim (1895), refers to solidarity and collective consciousness meaning that certain norms and mores are shared amongst groups of people. Therefore, implied within the concept of collective consciousness is the notion of a collective conscience. That is, people who share values also share a moral code. For Durkheim the increased division and specialisation of labour that he observed in the 19th century, and has intensified dramatically subsequently, would assist and depend on social solidarity. An 'organic' social system would be the result, and this form of society would for Durkheim be functional for both people and society notwithstanding an inevitable tension between individual freedom and the interdependence dependence of organic societal set-up.

The basis of social life Durkheim is altruism whereby individuals willingly participate in solidarity performances and forego self-interest for the collective good. He also pointed to how some dysfunctional societies or sub-sections of a society generate 'anomie'. Where society is not properly integrated because, for example, there are wide inequalities, violence, and insecurity, people may experience 'normlessness' and thereby suffer psychologically.

Wilde (2013) is in favour of 'radical humanism'. Radical humanism for him appreciates that there are universal human attributes including moral standards, reason and rationality, compassion, productiveness, and cooperation. Humans are capable of creativity, progressing intellectually, gaining pleasure from sex and play. Wilde argues that this approach demotes economic and technological forces and promotes social solidarity. I suggest social solidarity is paramount to the solving such social crisis as the climate emergency and economic and technological know-how needs to be harnessed to find suitable solutions. Wilde is also an advocate of possibilism, and it is possible to solve many if not all humanity's social crises.

The sociologist Amitai Etzioni (1993; 2014) promotes 'communitarianism' as a political philosophy with practical relevance to social solidarity in contemporary society. For example, Etzioni's communitarianism is the underlying ideology of the 'Third Way' policies of the UK's Labour governments during the 1990s and early 2000s. It also influenced governments and opposition political parties in the USA, the Netherlands, Germany, Sweden, and Denmark. For these governments, there was a need for an amalgamation of left-wing and right-wing politics that retained capitalism and centralism but would further egalitarianism and localism, and combine rights and responsibilities. State control and self-control would co-exist, as would personal freedom and community connectivity.

Communal Bystanding

Like kindness and cooperativeness counting when it comes to mental health, so does the community. The solidarity shown in social crises may at the outset seem surprising. As with kindness and cooperativeness, much of the cohesion and mutual support that bind communities all the world is hidden behind a wide screen of disharmony and indifference. People passing by or standing by rather than intervening when someone needs assistance after a road accident or robbery, and possibly being discouraged by other bystanders to not intervene, is considered a psychological phenomenon. The 'bystander effect' is a concept conceived by social psychologists John Darley and Bibb Latané (1968). In their social psychological laboratory experiments what these what these researchers observed is that intervention is affected by two factors, *'diffusion of responsibility' and 'social influence'. Diffusion of responsibility refers to the relationship between the decision by a bystander to act in an emergency and the number of other bystanders there are at the scene. The more bystanders the less likely anyone will take action. Personal responsibility becomes diffused amongst a crowd to the point where no individual feels she/he has the responsibility to intervene. Social influence* refers to how bystanders monitor the conduct and attitude of other bystanders. If one person seems to be initiating action, then others are more likely to follow. Equally, an individual perceives that no-one else is showing signs of intervening, then she/he will probably remain inactive.

It was the infamous murder of 28-year-old Kitty Genovese outside her apartment in New York City in 1964 that prompted these social psychologists to investigate why people don't get involved in emergency situations even when a life is at stake. This murder became infamous when it was reported in the press that dozens of neighbours had either seen the murder or heard the screams of the victim but had failed to help stop the perpetrator from continuing to stab his victim or to call the police. Eventually, one person did call the police, and although they arrived at the scene very quickly it was too late to save this young woman's life, and the attacker had fled although he was later arrested and convicted. However, the facts of this case and the notion that the bystander effect can be so potently nefarious has come into question by psychologist Rachel Manning and her colleagues (Manning *et al.*, 2007). The bystander effect does exist, they accept, but the story of Kitty Genovese' murder has become and urban myth and a misconstrued parable about human performance in psychology and social psychology textbooks. The facts of the case, they point out, were not that there were dozens of witnesses to the murder. They point to the Assistant District Attorney Charles Skoller's statement after the case that only about half a dozen witnesses had seen what was happening. Moreover, some of these witnesses reported that they didn't understand what was happening, with none of them admitting that they had seen the stabbing. One neighbour had shouted at the attacker to leave the woman alone and he had stooped the attack, only recompensing his attack in a nearby building which could not be overseen by the neighbours.

In emergency and non-emergency situations the bystander effect is affected by personal perceptions, individual skills, social conventions, and the context of the physical environment (Hammond, 2022). It may be unclear what is occurring, and this could lead to individual indecision about what the correct reaction should be or whether inaction is more appropriate. Individuals may feel they do not have the skills, for example, to carry-out life support techniques, or they cannot swim and therefore would drown themselves if they entered deep water to try to save someone else drowning. Cultural norms may mean that women are less prone to interfere with a man or the reverse may also be the case. There may not be relevant resources available such as a defibrillator or fire extinguisher, or connection to a mobile phone to call for help.

One other factor should be taken into consideration, and this applies to many laboratory-based psychological and social-psychological studies. Ethically, real 'experiments' measuring such phenomena as the bystander effect at murder scenes cannot take place let alone be replicated in order to demonstrate reliability. Hence, what is being offered by these laboratory experiments are either loose approximations or interesting insights regarding human performance. They may also lead to misunderstandings about how humans think, act, and behave, and some of these misunderstandings can lead to a vastly different impression of human nature and nurturing than that which supposes compassion, collegiality, and community are core to humanity's disposition.

A multitude of occurrences of social solidarity materialise during social crises. Some solidarity feats pre-exist the catastrophe in question but are then solidified *in extrēmīs*. Others are freshly distilled by disaster. A social crisis may have a particular type of solidarity. For example, the term 'pandemic solidary' is used by the activist collectively consisting of sociologist Marina Sitrin and the international group of writers called *Colectiva Semrara* to describe the phenomenon of individuals and communities coming together to provide mutual aid when COVID-19 became a major social crisis worldwide. These activists record a series of extant and emerging examples of social solidarity that survive when there is and isn't a social crisis the size of the COVID-19 pandemic (Sitrin and *Colectiva Semrara*, 2020).

For Sitrin and *Colectiva Semrara* social solidarity persists despite the principles and practices of capitalism operating antagonistically towards collective consciousness, a coalesced conscience, and catastrophes delivering destruction and death. That is, the orientation of an economic system towards commodification, consumerisation, and the idealising of the 'self', is in their view incompatible with the engendering communality, cooperativeness, and ethicality. Rather than securing solidarity, capitalism breeds inequality, alienation, and anomie.

Community and COVID-19

Moreover, the arrival of COVID-19 (and this applies to most social crises) might have been expected to have worsened the prospects of new forms of social solidarity developing and to have undone those existing already. But this did not happen argue Sitrin and her colleagues. Social solidarity not only survived but prospered. They provide examples of social solidarity during the COVID-19 pandemic are provided from Syria, Turkey, Iraq, Taiwan, South Korea, India, Mozambique, Zimbabwe, South Africa, Portugal, Greece, Italy, the UK, Turtle Island (Canada), Argentina, and Brazil. For these activists, abundant instances of solidarity are happening every day across the world. These include families working together, work colleagues collaborating, and toiling of non-government, charitable and religious organisations to improve the lives of disadvantaged if not endangered individuals. Moreover, they contend that there is furtherance of kindness and heroics when disasters strike and did so during the COVID-19 pandemic.

Political Solidarity

However, scholar of ethics in Medicine Ruud ter Meulen (2017), questions whether the notion of social solidarity is out-of-date, a vestige of Christian and communist idealism. He asks, Is individualism that is concomitant with consumerism, commodification, not the more realistic appraisal of human performance in the 21st century? However, Meulen reasons that individuality and social solidity are not necessarily contradictory or dysfunctional facets of the contemporary societal system. Respecting individuality can coincide with an overarching moral, legal, and political framework that promotes justice and protects the vulnerable. That is, the adherence to social rules and norms that confine exploitation and neglect (at least in their excessive configurations) while giving licence to individual agency, is possible. Indeed, managing this balance is what socially liberal and democratic governments along with their related institutions struggle with constantly. Balancing social solidarity and individual agency are the fundamentals of the social contract between the powerful and privileged and the rest of the population in these societal formations, at least on superficial analysis. This struggle is manifest within countries ruled by authoritarian governments or dictators and their citizens, as well as between those countries and much of the rest of the world that has either already adopted is in the process of adopting 'global capitalism'. But one implication of the questions raised by Meulen is that social solidarity can become overbearing if not repressive. There is a historical president for this outcome.

Soviet Russia is one example where policies were introduced for the 'good of society' (or more accurately, for the good of the State and its senior operatives). Not long after the Bolshevik revolution, Soviet ideologues and their propagandists introduced the notion of 'The New Man' or *Homo Sovieticus* (Zinoviev, 1986). The notion of a new Soviet Woman was based on the old pre-Soviet woman as subservient to men, but now also to the State. Amongst the core the characteristics advocated for this reconstructed individual were to be selflessness, self-mastery, diligence, and an enthusiasm for spreading Soviet-style communism, not driven by innate and unconscious impulses (which for the connoisseurs of communist publicity were fictions of Western psychology). What would drive The New Man would be a raised consciousness that put the good of the collective above that on the individual.

Social and medical anthropologist Iza Kavedžija (2022) concludes from her investigations into communal living in different cultural settings that there are lessons to be learned about how people in the rest of society could improve their lives. Kavedžija affirms the positions that are also some of the staple positions presented in this book. She argues that somatic and mental unwellness and well-being are the outcome of societal situations, and people need solid and suitable social connections to thrive both physically and psychologically. Bad societal situations and bad social connections are detrimental to the mind and body. Kavedžija's review of anthropological studies leads her to promote the idea that living together if done well, not only works for the benefit of the individual but for the Common good. What she is alluding to is that the Soviet-style of 'living together' whereby the needs of the collective must prioritise those of the individual is not an inevitability.

Conviviality and Community

Kavedžija focuses on the importance of conviviality and care in communities. She defines conviviality as the art of living well together. She extracts from the anthropological studies in her investigation what she sees as a common thread, and this is that people living in small communities strive to improve their environmental and relationships when the State and formal organisations have a negligible role in their lives. Kavedžija provides the example of traditional Amazonian communities in which caring is reified through the sharing of resources, and emotional stability is cultivated through a much more relaxed lifestyle that is the norm in South American urban conurbations. She also offers the example of the traditional Japanese habit of neighbourhood communal bathing that also served as places for family members and friends to socialise and embed social connections.

Communal living should, suggests, Kavedžija, encompass conviviality with other species. Humans share the earth with animals, including internal microbes, and plants. But presently, that space is not being shared for the common good of all species, and the dominant genus (Homo sapiens) is not even capable as yet of making the space convivial for itself due to an imbalance it has created with these other species. Furthermore, humans today share their world with increasingly complicated technologies, which are becoming more 'artificially intelligent'. Artificial intelligence for humanity could turn out to be 'modern magic' or hold a 'dangerous Future' (Wilks, 2019). If the latter, then added to humanity's un-convivial dominance over other species will be an un-convivial relationship with artificial intelligence. Historian Yuval Harari (2017) warns that humanity is profoundly ill-prepared to deal with future technology. In particular, humans are ignoring the impending influence of artificial intelligence which Harari suggests will transform the global economy, culture, and politics. It may also alter bodies and minds to-date unimaginable ways Forces not yet known from artificial intelligence, and algorithmic control of 'dig data', robotic automation, biotechnology, genetic engineering, and nanoscience, may manufacture a world that is not convivial to human dominance or existence. In the meantime, these technologies may add to human psychological suffering or sooth that suffering by means of yet to be comprehended 'modern magic'.

It is wrong to situate, contends Kavedžija, the cause of emotional distress within the individual. For example, the extensive coverage of 'bad news' is not good for mental health:

> It is not inconceivable that our current mental health crisis is intertwined with our witnessing of large-scale suffering and neglect of humans, nonhumans and the natural world.
>
> (Kavedžija, 2022)

Kavedžija proposes that personal resources such as resilience are not formulated from only within the individual. They arise from the positive interchanges with other people, and from the emotionally uplifting and validating values generated from socially solid communities. Just as kindness is contagious so is optimism. Hopefulness is all the more possible if receiving signals of hope from those with whom one is cultivating a communal lifestyle.

Commonality of Communities

Communities are everywhere all the time. Formal and informal local lobby groups, friendship groups, hobby groups, sports groups, extended family networks, and work-based networks, are but a few examples of interpersonal connectivity beyond personal partnerships and immediate family memberships. The internet has an alienating, atomising, and abusive, side but also a side that allows and enhances communities. These communities may be geographically provincial, national, international, or global. Social media and online-meeting facilities such as 'Zoom' have revolutionised interpersonal and inter-agency bonding.

The position that there is a real rise in psychological suffering worldwide may induce more than a plea for even more attention to be focused on fixing faults in the individual. For example, researchers from the National Institute of Mental Health, the primary agency of the US government responsible for biomedical and health-related research, support a 'whole-of-society' approach to deal with what they, among many others (see Chapter 2) assert is a mental health crisis (Rahman *et al.*, 2020). As part of that approach, and following a lead from the United Nations, the National Institute of Mental Health has supported the setting-up of 'global research hubs' in low- and middle-income countries. These hubs are designed to deliver rapid mental health services that are interdisciplinary, sustainable, and based on robust empirical evidence. They also have a commitment to bring together representativeness from the governmental, non-governmental agencies, and the local community. Examples of these hubs are cited from Pakistan, Uganda, Sierra Leone, India, Thailand, Mozambique, and Columbia. Evidence-based policies and practices are utilised by community health workers to deal with, for example, children with disruptive behaviours, psychological effects from involvement in warfare, and suicide amongst farmers, and at the time when COVID-19 was spreading globally, helping to alleviate 'pandemic anxiety' amongst children and support front-line workers. These hubs, therefore, can be considered to help solidify communities because they are combining generalised knowledge with a local means of implementing that knowledge. However, the passing on of external expertise (which is what 'evidence-based' practice entails) to manage internal issues (in both senses of that term) doesn't necessarily underscore community solidarity. The demarcation between local and generalised knowledge is widened further when the latter emanates in the main from Western countries and is advocated by national and supra-national agencies rather than by the community concerned. These hubs are at root a top-down innovation rather than bottom-up, and as such may not be 'owned' by the community.

Historian Fay Alberti (2020) notes that the COVID-19 pandemic's negative aspects such as loneliness can be balanced with and possibly outweighed by positive happenings, and the latter is significant because it is both surprising and profound:

> [W]e are seeing some positive and unexpected results, including widespread outpourings of charity, togetherness and empathy for complete strangers. We might even be seeing a grassroots redefinition of what "community" means in the 21st century.
>
> (Alberti, 2020)

For Alberti, the COVID-19 pandemic revitalised the concept of community and revitalised the actuality of community. But I suggest that community did not need to be revitalised or actualised. It has never gone away. Social Crises inspire novel kinds of conjoint human performances, but they do not invent mutuality. That said, Alberti's sampling of human cooperation, kindness, and community are worth mentioning to show some of the novel ways in which people helped each other and did so not for money or an elevation of status.

At the time of writing, the debate continues about whether the virus SARS-CoV-2 originated in the Wuhan wet-market or the nearby research laboratory (BBC News, 2023). No matter whether market or laboratory (although the weight of evidence indicates it was the former), this Chinese city remains the focus of the outbreak and of the consequential isolation measures enforced strictly by the Chinese Government. But for Alberti Wuhan also exemplifies mutuality. Despite the perceived dangers volunteers stepped forward to give lifts in their cars so that health and care workers could get to work. In the USA, where there were mixed messages about risks from the disease and even doubts about its existence by some of the most politically powerful people in the country, some of the least powerful took it upon themselves to act. Alberti mentions the First Nation Americans who set up a helpline to organise the supply of personal protection equipment for hospital workers in New York. Another example given by Alberti is how thousands of volunteers in Canada gave food to vulnerable people, including impoverished international students. Yet another example comes from Brazil where volunteers provided food to people living in slums. In the UK during the early stages of the pandemic, millions of people volunteered when asked by the Government and charities to support people who were not able to collect groceries or medicines, were lonely, or who were emotionally distressed some of whom had a diagnosis of mental disorder. Millions of UK citizens also came to the front of their houses to 'clap' at a time set by the Government in support of front-line workers, especially health and social care workers. There is also an indication that people in that country sensed that community ties had been strengthened and society overall had become kinder (Legal and General, 2020).

Alberti concludes with the observation that although some or all of the types of community action particular to a social crisis such as COVID-19 may subside or disappear when it resolves, these examples demonstrate the very essence of the meaning of 'community', a term that for her has become so overused as to be meaningless. To be meaningful, suggests Alberti, community must encompass more than a shared interest. There has to be a positive psychological payoff for participants, and this has to build personal and social resilience. Participants must be committed to the common good and, in turn, that does them good.

However, the distribution of community togetherness and kindness may be unequal, and reversible. There is some evidence that rather than 'coming together' the COVID-19 pandemic there was a degree of 'coming apart'. Although there was a resurgence of neighbourliness, local cohesion may have been weakened by the negative effects of the pandemic on physical and mental health caused by financial and employment security, and social isolation. There also the suggestion that cultural and structural seeds need to be in place for community support to prosper when a social crisis like the COVID-19 pandemic arrives. In vulnerable communities these seeds may not be present or if present their growth is inhibited by a barrier of poverty, ill-health, and discrimination (Borkowska and Laurence, 2021).

Ian Goldin, scholar of globalisation and technological and economic development, is adamant that there is such a phenomenon as 'society' rather than a collection of individuals, and that individual selfishness has not displaced social solidary, and that. He refers to events occurring when the COVID-19 pandemic. For him there was an outpouring of solidarity:

> The young sacrificed their social lives, education and jobs and took on enormous debts to help the elderly….. Essential workers placed themselves at daily risk to staff our care homes and hospitals and ensure food was delivered, rubbish collected and the lights stayed on.
>
> (Goldin, 2021, p.224)

Goldin adds that many people sacrificed their own health to help others to survive the pandemic. Many carried their life-saving tasks anonymously, although groups such as health workers were hailed as heroes (Goldin, 2021). Although the attribution was not constantly applied, other heroes of the COVID-19 identified by the public, politicians, and the press, were the police, pharmacists, farm workers, grocers, and garbage collectors. If not applauded (literally at times in the UK) as heroes, then these groups were considered as 'essential workers'.

The COVID-19 Social Study Report referred to in Chapter 2 focuses on the negative impact of the pandemic (Fancourt *et al.*, 2022). What is also mentioned are caveats revealing positive effects, but not with the same degree of emphasis as the pandemic's harmful consequences. Specifically, mention is made of displays of communality and compliance. From an alternative perspective (complementing the one taken in this book), the following observation from the two-year study of one of the worst social crises faced not just by the UK but the world since the two world wars should have been far more prominent in such an important and comprehensive research project:

> [T]he vast majority of people acted for the common good, volunteering for their communities, feeling connected to the values of their neighbourhoods, and maintaining high compliance rates throughout the pandemic… Behavioural fatigue, selfish behaviours, and rule breaking were very much in the minority….
>
> (Fancourt *et al.*, 2022, p.73)

The finding that the performance of most people for the most part from the most serious dislocation of everyday life and of societal systems, and most serious threat to physical and psychological well-being and to personal survival, is so remarkable that it should be celebrated and circulated to the same degree if not more so than the negative psychological and social consequences. That said, the researchers responsible for the COVID-19 Social Study do make recommendations that include extensive governmental and community collaboration aimed at fostering social solidarity and cohesion.

Community and Environment

The physical environment fuses with the social environment and in their combined condition they affect mental health positively or negatively. Bustling, densely populated, noxious, and noisome environments, are not noted for engendering psychological serenity. A becalmed built milieu is more likely to becalm the mind (Halpern, 2013). Disasters do not usually engender tranquillity. But pandemic disasters may well be unique compared with other disasters because of lockdowns. According to Goldin (2021), for the first time in centuries, much of the world became static. Lockdowns calm the industrial, trade, travel, work, leisure, and schooling commotion of typical society. The reduction or cessation of the flow of traffic and the multitudinous interconnecting activities of retailing, manufacturing, and education, becalmed the physical environment. This becalming of the physical environment had direct benefits for society including a reduction in air pollution, unrecyclable waste, and traffic accidents. The transmission of the extant infectious disease also reduces significantly during lockdowns and outside those periods but when cross-infection control measures were followed by large swathes of populations (Brueggemann *et al.*, 2021).

Lockdowns also directly benefit people. The calming of society enforces a slower, less pressurised pace of life. More time becomes available for hobbies, exercise, and family interactions. They also provide opportunities to enhance social solidarity. Simply having the time and 'head space' to say hello to a neighbour or even a stranger is socially solidifying. A study conducted in the

Spanish province of Tarragona found that the number of traffic accidents dropped by nearly 75% during the period of a lockdown lasting from 16 March to 26 April 2020 (Saladié *et al.*, 2020). The global response to the COVID-19 pandemic has driven the biggest annual fall in CO_2 emissions since the Second World War, a reduction of 7% (Friedlingstein *et al.*, 2020). When lockdowns were imposed more people undertook more walks in outdoor public places and time spent more time in their gardens. Of course, this mainly applied to those who had easy access to those green spaces and owned gardens (Sandhu, 2021). However, the personal positives are offset by the psychological commotion caused by concerns over contracting the virus, losing love-ones, and becoming unemployed (although some governments implemented policies to save jobs). The societal negatives are the commotion caused to the economy, businesses, and health systems.

Another surprising consequence of the COVID-19 pandemic has been that despite an initial frenzy of consumption, much of which took place via the internet, there are indications that overall people became less materialistic There was, although again relatively short-lived, questioning of lifestyles and search for more meaningful ways of living life than accumulating more and more money-driven status and 'things' (Andrés, 2022).

Layla McCay is a psychiatrist who specialises in mental health and urban design. Todd Litman specialises in transportation technologies and services and how they may affect people and communities. Jenny Roe is a landscape architect and environmental psychologist. Together they have published a wealth of research and ideas on how to design urban environments to support and improve the mental well-being of the inhabitants (Litman, 2021; 2022; McCay and Litman, 2021; McCay and Roe, 2021; Roe and McCay, 2021). Collectively, the work of these scholars points to the need to recognise the importance of the physical environment to mental health. For example, the COVID-19 pandemic stranded whole populations either in their houses or in their neighbourhood for long periods. Those with spacious living arrangements and gardens, and who lived in high-quality local areas, perhaps with nearby parks and shops, were in a better position to maintain emotional fortitude than those residing in overcrowded conditions without adjacent amenities. These scholars also point out that the opportunity to partake in physical exercise enhances both physical and mental well-being. Moreover, they posit that good spatial features reduce the incidence of anxiety, depression, and suicide, and foster trust and empathy.

How cities are built, therefore, is a crucial factor for sustaining psychological and social solidity in world where most people have moved into urban environments. However, Litman, McCay, and Roe recognise that the causative connection between the urban environment and psychological suffering is complex. There are overriding confounding factors including poverty. Moreover, it could be there is a reverse in the cause-and-effect relationship. That is, 'social drift' may be occurring whereby impoverished people already suffering from or vulnerable to emotional distress move into cities.

Wars are not noted for engendering quietness. But Bregman (2020) quotes medical practitioner John MacCurdy (1943) who in October drove through a poor part of London following the severe bombing of that are by the German Luftwaffe. MaCurdy notes not panic and mayhem but a serenity. Despite the craters and crumbling buildings people were composed and getting on with everyday living as best as they could amongst the rubble. Far from riots and raiding, children played, adults shopped, and policemen directed traffic.

Scientific Solidarity

Yet another surprise is how science as opposed to nonsense prevailed throughout the COVID-19 pandemic. Technological and intellectual endeavour and accomplishments did exist alongside vacuous conjecture and insolvent conniving as well as legitimate criticism of scientific knowledge during social crises and non-crises times. But, veracity, integrity, facts, and science have made a comeback. Post-modernism, social constructionism, cultural relativity, post-truth, fake-news and fake-news about fake-news, and downright lies, although present were laid low, or had to compromise. While dissembling, dishonesty, and conspiracy theories have proliferated (especially on the internet) during the pandemic, the public presence of science has increased more so (Fonseca *et al.*, 2023).

However, the social standing of science in normal times is equivocal. There is good and bad science, including good and bad pharmacology. The academic writings of general practitioner Ben Goldacre (2009; 2012; 2014) is relevant here especially regarding the scientific 'miracle' of COVID-19 vaccines (McKie, 2020). Mathematician Hannah Fry and geneticist Adam Rutherford (2021) admits that science is biased. The bias is towards publishing dramatic, novel, and positive, results. The sociological concept of scientism (Morrall, 2009) typifies science as belief system in which scientific knowledge is considered supreme over other ways of understanding the world. But Goldacre (2009) believes fervently in 'good' science. But Goldacre accepts there is a lot of 'bad' science that is presented by its originators or is presented by others, either naively or with deceitful intention, as evidence of authentic scholarship.

But the apparent robustness of empirical evidence about the characteristics of this virus, self and societal protection, treatment, and prevention, has upgraded the societal significance of science. An outstanding example of good science is the development of COVID-19 vaccines. Other outstanding scientific successes in 2020 include using artificial intelligence to solve how proteins fold into three-dimensional shapes which has implications for the treatment of multiple diseases (DeepMind, 2020).

Scientists and their research hit the headlines throughout the COVID-19 pandemic. They were presented each day in the media as the authoritative discourse on disease and how whole populations and whole countries if not the world should operate (Goldin, 2021). Scientists and experts have had their status restored and, after some being the object of political disdain are being taken seriously again and informing policies, albeit at the risk of being manipulated and blamed when things go wrong.

> The global health and economic crisis has highlighted the need for interdisciplinary expertise, with the roles of behavioural and economic sciences being as vital as that of medical expertise in weighing up the costs and benefits of different measures.
>
> (Goldin, 2021, p.249)

Medical sciences, economics, psychology, social psychology, anthropology, and sociology amongst many other disciplines contributed to the revealing and remedying of COVID-19 as they have or could to the understanding and allaying if not hindrance of other social crises.

> 2020 is likely to go down in history as a watershed year in scientific advancement.
>
> (Goldin, 2021, p.250)

During 2020 Vaccinologist Sarah Gilbert and biologist Catherine Green, along with many colleagues at Oxford University, in allied agencies, and at the pharmaceutical company Astra Zeneca, fashioned and furnished a vaccine against COVID-19. They did this in record time. Their work saved millions of lives and protected billions of people from a debilitating disease (Gilbert and Green, 2022).

Gilbert and Green note that within hours of announcing that they were recruiting volunteers for their vaccine trials, thousands of people had applied. They comment that they were humbled by this level of altruism and how it reinforced their belief that people are in the main good and generous (Gilbert and Green, 2022). Gilbert and Green also record the high degree of international cooperation and creative ideas they had from other academics and members of the bioscience industry. They refer to the enormous goodwill and industriousness displayed by the teams working directly on the development of the vaccine. Astra Zeneca's top-level personnel also contributed to the general unselfishness by deciding to manufacture the vaccine at cost while the pandemic lasted and to continue to do so for poor countries.

Gilbert and Green write that going back to pre-pandemic normality is not to be recommended. During the pandemic, Science and scientists have become more respected despite the plague of misinformation that spread employment practices and the life-work balance became refashioned beneficently, and a colossal boost to volunteering. But the pandemic affected negatively maternal and new-born health, gender and racial equality, mental health, routine health monitoring, and early diagnosis and treatment of other life-threatening diseases such as cancer and increased the wealth divide.

Ironically, science, so far, has not served psychiatry well. Notwithstanding the considerable connectedness of psychiatry (and to a lesser but growing extent, psychology, and psychotherapy) to the neurosciences, endocrinology, immunology, and cognitive sciences, few successes can be claimed without contradiction. But nonsense serves the psyche even less well.

Coping and Hoping

In March 2020 a sociological study based at Swansea University in the UK and named 'The CoronaDiaries Project' began to collect first-hand reports about how people were managing their lives during the COVID-19 pandemic (Michael Ward,[2] 2022). The project over two years obtained nearly 1,000 submissions from 184 participants between 11 and 89 years of age living in 14 different countries. The submissions came in the form of, for example, notebooks, diaries, videos, social media postings, photographs, songs, poems, shopping lists, artwork, and music playlists. They contained accounts of catching and surviving the disease, losing loved ones, and loneliness and isolation particularly during 'lockdowns' when interpersonal contact was curtailed or ceased. But what is also revealed in the accounts is how quickly people adapted to the crisis and displayed elements of creativity, humour, and resilience.

Resilience as a Contentious Concept

Resilience is the ability to cope with the normal stress of life as well as being able to deal with traumatic events (Nieuwerburgh and Nacif, 2020). Epidemiologists Emily Goldmann and Sandro Galea (2014) reveal that most people who experience a traumatic event do not develop psychopathology. What is more common is adaptation to these circumstances. People quickly learn to cope. However, that personal resilience does necessarily result in an absence of some degree of psychological suffering.

Resilience as a concept and as a personal requirement, if a crisis is to be overcome, is controversial. There is an evolving definition when it comes to resilience. According to the American Psychological Association (APA) resilience is defined as the process of adapting well in the face of trauma or tragedy, threats or other significant sources of stress (Southwick *et al.*, 2014). Resilience is exists on a continuum and is applicable to multiple personal and societal domains (Southwick *et al.*, 2014).

The promotion of resilience as a beneficial human quality has a downside and may be irrelevant in some situations. For example, academic success depends on other factors such as attendance and study habits rather than only on resilience. When resilience is promoted in workplaces as an ideal to which workers should aspire this can conceal genuine difficulties in an individual's ability to handle stress caused by organisation malfunctions rather than personal malfunctioning. For moral responsibility and political theorist Katy Dineen (2020), the promotion hope is a better alternative to resilience. Dineen defines hope as the capacity for an individual to identify meaningful goals, and to have the motivation to attain them. There is therefore a difference between hope and resilience, suggests Dineen. Resilience is not about change whereas the outcome of hope is intended to be change. Ilan Kelman (2020; 2021) is a specialist in disasters and health. Kelman is clear that 'natural' disasters' are due to societal failures and concurs with Dineen that advocating personal resilience should be about change. Kelman, however, considers resilience as a quality that can incorporate change, and that change needs to be about improving society.

Coping with Wars and Nuclear Catastrophes

Sociologist Charles Fritz (1996; original 1961) argues that far from psycho-pathology large-scale disasters produce what he refers to as 'mentally healthy conditions'. Moreover, societal resilience, in the main, overcomes any weakness in societal systems and structures:

> Nations and communities typically demonstrate amazing toughness and resiliency in absorbing and coping with the disintegrative effects of disaster. And disaster-struck societies not only quickly rebound from disaster but often reconstruct and regenerate their social life with added increments of vitality and productivity.
>
> (Fritz, 1996, p.32)

Disasters are, accepts Fritz, events that can cause profound human misery. The death and destruction they produce may elicit great suffering among the survivors. But Fritz argues that the preoccupation with these physical effects and corresponding psychological problems means the positive consequences of disaster for surviving individuals, communities, and society are frequently overlooked. Most of the personal and societal pathologies of normal times fail to rise and may decline in disaster. Countries and communities tend not to disintegrate but demonstrate both personal and societal resilience and regeneration when affected by disaster.

The normal routines, rules, and responsibilities of individuals and societies are shaken, and many are either entirely ended or firmly re-affirmed. Novel and persistent cultural customs enable personal and societal innovation and are given added impetus out of urgent necessity. These imperatives are mostly achievable, points out Fritz, without intervention from the psychiatric, psychological, psychotherapy, and psychopharmacological disciplines. Disaster provides a stark contrast to the mundanities, trivialities, and boredom of everyday existence. Surviving and sorting seriously sinister, scary, and scarring situations, if survived, can be invigorating; membership in what Fritz refers to as a 'community of suffers' also offers a unique form of social support:

> *The widespread sharing of danger, loss, and deprivation produces an intimate, primarily group solidarity among the survivors which overcomes social isolation, provides a channel for intimate communication and expression, and provides a major source of physical and emotional support and reassurance.* [italics in original]
>
> (Fritz, 1996, p.84)

Fritz is aware that his observations are not definitive either in terms of his analysis of them or as incontrovertible conclusions. But Fritz has come to his conclusion disasters are not necessarily destructive or damaging to the mental health of victims. The development of these ideas gradually emerged from personal and research experiences covering a period of about 18 years from 1943 to 1962. These experiences are as follows:

- As a participant-observer in wartime England from 1943 to 1946
- As a Staff Member of the U.S. Strategic Bombing Survey from 1945 to 1946
- As Associate Director of the Disaster Project, National Opinion Research Center, University of Chicago, from 1950 to 1954
- As Research Associate, Committee on Disaster Studies and Assistant Director, Disaster Research Group, National
- Academy of Sciences-National Research Council, Washington, DC, from 1954 to 1959
- As Associate Professor, Department of Psychiatry, College of Medicine, and Director of the College's Behavioral Science, Division, University of Florida, Gainesville, Florida, from 1959 to 1962

It is Fritz's wartime experience as a, in his terms, 'participant observer', that seems to have influenced him the most. By 1943, observe Fritz, the British had already endured five years of war. Their cities had been bombed, and they were undergoing severe shortages of shelter, food, clothing, and public services. Under those conditions, points out Fritz, it might be expected that the population would be demoralised, weary, and in a state of perpetual anxiety. But this is not what happened, according to Fritz. What Fritz says he observed was a nation of 'gloriously happy people', with an increase in social interactions between and within socially different groupings, especially in the bars. Fritz refers also to the 'great resilience' of the defeated nations in the Second World War, with both Germany and Japan rebounding from devastation to become economic powerhouses.

Medical practitioner Radha Modgil notes:

> We often don't realise just how courageous and resilient we are being, or how incredible we are in the midst of all this. We can't, or don't, see ourselves for who we truly are or who we are becoming through adversity.
>
> (Modgil, 2021)

But sociologist Eve Passerini (2000) highlights contradictory results from studies on disaster recovery and reconstruction. Some studies that show social change is unlikely after disasters; some show that change occurs frequently after disasters, and others show that both can occur concurrently. For

Passerini, the solidarity, openness, and change in norms, that often emerge in the early stages of disaster recovery can be fragile and short-lived. That said, Passerini finds that most studies do not show any evidence of long-term psychological effects and physical infrastructure is usually rebuilt without much change from the original.

Medical practitioner and public health researcher Nikunj Makwana (2019) examines what she determines are the 'protective factors' for mental health in disaster situations. She does suggest the need for programs aimed at informing vulnerable populations about the negative effects on mental health from disaster and how to handle these and implementing policies for 'maintaining harmony in the environment' and 'creating social and economic well-being' when disaster strikes (that is, ensuring resources necessary for survival are not only available but distributed fairly). However, Makwana focuses mainly on the personal resources of the individual. For her, those individuals with an ability and alacrity to control emotional extremes and are endowed with optimism, and audacity, have regard for their own safety and that of others, accept their circumstances and are prepared to deal with the fallout from the disaster, are less likely to suffer from mental debilitation. These attributes are for Makwana encapsulated under the key personal resource of 'resilience'.

Resilience for Makwana is central to the ethos of 'positive psychology', and its benefit for the individual is how it promotes physical, social, and emotional protectiveness and thereby enhances significantly that person's quality of life. There is, acknowledges Makwana, a social side to resilience in the sense of resilient communities. Personal resilience for Makwana is the ability to deal effectively with 'negative situations' combined with the ability to recover instantly and to be able to prepare for potential future calamities. Social resilience proses Makwana, is when there are inherent structures and systems within the community that help to avert disasters or diminish their effects. Makwana's proposition replicates the stance of Goldmann and Galea (2014). Survival for people and their communities is made more possible, adds Makwana when the attributes of resilience are found in both. These attributes, however, are contradictory. Those people who value their own individuality and are more insistent on self-help and communities that are cohesive and inclusive (especially if there is common religious belief) argues Makwana, are more effective in coping with the aversive provocations on their lives and infrastructures brought about by the tragedies of terrorist attacks.

To repeat, most people facing a social crisis cope. The ability to cope may have emanated from the individual's or her/his community's forerunning capacities or with the facilitation of outside help from other communities, aid workers, and a range of professionals offering practical and psychological support. The latter may take the form of trauma therapy, mindfulness, or one form or another of cognitive-behavioural therapy. Regarding the latter, any psychotherapeutic intervention may not reap resilience to any more than a modest extent, and some may be counterproductive. Indeed, at a community level, measures intended to reduce exposure to radioactivity after a disaster may also be counterproductive, producing an increase in anxiety.

Even in the case of a nuclear catastrophe people may demonstrate resilience rather than resignation. For example, the pregnant residents and families with young children living near the Three Mile Island power plant radiation leak occurred were given contradictory advice about whether to evacuate. Not only did the inconsistency in information generate fear, but raising the issue of the threat of radioactive contamination contributed to an intensification of fearfulness. There would seem to be no evidence of physiological harm to residents from the leak at Three Mile Island, but the reputed danger did supplement the pool of factors associated with disasters that are psychologically destabilising (Longmuir and Agyapon, 2022).

Below the Pacific Ocean, about 80 miles from the city of Sendai in the Tohoku region of the Japanese island of Honshu, and massive earthquake erupted. The earthquake caused a Tsunami. The damage from 40 feet waves when it hit the island resulted in approximately 15,000 of deaths and hundreds of thousands of people being made homeless, the ruin of hundreds of businesses and the destruction of much of the area's road and railway infrastructure. Even more problematic in terms of the tsunami's devastating impact was the flooding and meltdown of three nuclear reactors at the Fukushima Daiichi Nuclear power plant and the release of radioactivity. More than 150,000 people had to be evacuated (Kobayashi *et al.*, 2022). Some of the elderly and those who were moved out of hospitals died during the evacuation (Longmuir and Agyapon, 2022).

Similar to what happened in Three Mile Island, there were no credible reports of physical harm caused by the radiation leakage from the Fukushima Daiichi nuclear accident. Also, like Three Mile Island, however, was an elevated fear of contamination among residents. 'Radiation anxiety' resulted in worries about the possibility that houses, the land, and food had become adulterated. Contributing to the anxiousness of the local population was the stigma they attracted due to the fear of others that the evacuees might be radioactive.

Wars that spread worldwide are social crises of such disastrous magnitude that they seem to bear no comparison in terms of loss of life, and the disastrous disruption to economic and cultural edifices, routines, and norms. There are two potential crises that would surpass the ruination of previous world wars. The first if there was a nuclear disaster of global proportions, either started intentionally or unintentionally. The second is the climate emergency. Both disasters pose the risk of extinguishing humanity and most if not all other life forms.

But even the previous world wars and nuclear bombings and accidents have produced paradoxes. Disaster and progress can and frequently cohabit in the same historical space. Disaster is manifest and measurable. It is the tens of millions of people who die and the hundreds of millions who are physically and psychologically injured. It is the disruption and destruction of communities if not whole nations, the way of life for billions of people, property, land, sanitation systems, the production and distribution of supply food and water, and the family configuration (families were depleted of male adults due to the killing). Many countries are left with enormous financial debt or unpayable reparations (the latter happened to Germany after the First World War).

Wars that spread worldwide are social crises of such disastrous magnitude global society can be described as having gone insane. But wars that spread worldwide also furnish society with unsurpassed sanities although these may not occur until the insanity abates and unfortunately may eventually regress into their former states. Progress through the world being at war (although not every nation was actively involved, all were affected by the fighting) has occurred in science, medicine, education, housing, provision, and human rights, in general, and the rights of women, in particular. Mass bombing meant that once hostilities had ended there was revamping or replacing of much of the infrastructure needed for transport, water supply, sewage disposal, and food production, and accommodation.

The antecedents of some of these progressive changes existed before both the First World War and the Second World War so they may have happened without the need for devastation to be the catalyst. But these colossal conflicts altered and accelerated their trajectories.

> The Second World War (WWII) was one of the major transformative events of the 20th century…
>
> (Kesternich *et al.*, 2014)

There is irony, however, about which countries benefitted the most economically. By the late 1980s the countries that had lost the Second World War in military terms, Germany, Japan, and Italy, had higher per capita economic growth that the victorious countries except for the USA (Kesternich *et al.*, 2014). Also, the infrastructure of two of the losing countries benefited more in the long term. So much of Germany's infrastructure had been destroyed by the bombing raids of the allies, it could be modernised (with the aid enormous financial assistance from the 'Marshal Plan' set up by USA President Truman in 1948), whereas the UK remains with much of what was laid down in the Victorian era.

Between 60 and 80 million people are estimated to have died due to the Second World War. The civilian death toll was very high compared with the First World War, probably half of the overall number of fatalities. About ten million civilians were murdered for their political or religious belief, sexual preference, mental/brain condition, and ethnic, or economic identity (Kesternich *et al.*, 2014).

> During the twentieth century the world experienced two deadly global wars followed by a 'cold war' of unparallel expense and danger. World War 1 opened this brutal epoch.
>
> (Broadberry and Harrison, 2005, p.1)

A study of survivors of the atom bombs dropped on Hiroshima and Nagasaki, who then was living in the USA (65 years later), by Nurse researcher Amy Knowles using what she describes as a 'holistic health perspective' revealed aspects of suffering and thriving. For Knowles (2011), suffering and thriving for the subjects of her study are not separate states but exist on a fluid and time continuum. Where an individual is on that continuum varies over time. Some individuals may stay at or near one point indefinitely. Resilience as a personal trait acts on suffering and thriving as an intermediary 'lever'. Movement towards either suffering or thriving depends on the operation of this lever.

> Resilience serves as a lever, allowing individuals to move from one area to another as events or situations arise. When resilience is high, an individual will exhibit traits of thriving. Conversely, if the level of resilience drops, the person will move down into survival mode.
>
> (Knowles, 2011, pp.58–59)

However, there is conceptual overlap between surviving, thriving, and resilience. There is no universally agreed definition of resilience (Vella and Pai, 2019). It is applied to many different scenarios and used by very different clinical and academic disciplines. A further definitional snag is a need to consider whether personal and societal elements can be separated or are unavoidably and unalterably interlinked. To achieve definition accuracy consideration also needs to be given to the issue of whether resilience has an innate or learned pedigree. Knowles give what she designates as a broad definition of resilience. For her resilience is the positive adjustment in the face of adversity.

But 'positive adjustment' in the 'face of adversity' suggests that they are thriving having survived. That is, resilience implies both surviving and thriving. Therefore, to present resilience as a lever acting 'on' survival and thriving is not only oxymoronic but teleological and detracts from the useful insights provided by Knowles. Given that both surviving and thriving in the way these terms are used by Knowles imply survival, in order to delineate these states of human performance more suitable descriptors are 'coping' and 'hoping'.

The insights provided by Knowles include how individuals who were in a state of surviving rather than thriving, at the time of the research, exhibited anxiety about their own health and the health of another member of their family. The worry over health would be triggered whenever they or a family member suffered a minor illness because it was feared she/he would be vulnerable to more serious illnesses having possibly been contaminated by radiation or that future generations would inherit genetic disorders. These anxious individuals were also mistrustful, experienced feelings of stigma, and tended towards looking reflecting pessimistically on the past rather than having an optimistic view of the present and prospective lives. Their worrying carried a 'significant psychological burden' that undermined their capacity to thrive. Those Knowles places in the category of 'thriving', apart from not displaying any or much negativity such as suspiciousness and shamefulness, they showed forgiveness, and were actively involved in social campaigns such as the peace movement, and in animal welfare.

Knowles infers that thriving is innate, possibly an evolutionary trait, but does so without any robust data or rigorous theorising to back support these contentions. Promoting a biological basis for thriving risks accentuates and gives credence to the negativity Knowles found in her research subjects. It is to imply that hoping is hopeless and that coping is all that can be counted on in their lives. This negative perspective on the foundation of human performance is challenged implicitly and explicitly throughout this book. It is worth repeating that both nature and nurture matter to a greater or lesser extent to the formation and development of human thinking, feeling, and acting. Regarding continuing after catastrophe, personal and societal positivity is possible. Contrarily, comments that there is a connection between resilience and culture. She refers to how for some of the survivors, the strong family ties and stability found in traditional Japanese culture fostered resilience. Knowles also appreciates how resilience is affected by culturally based health beliefs, access to resources, and previous experience with hardship.

It is important to recognise, however, that some of the survivors of the atomic bombing of their cities had debilitating injuries and diseases. These injuries and diseases debilitated psychological reclamation let alone psychological regeneration. Returning to a previous way of viewing the world, on whatever part of the Knowles' continuum this may have been, would have been difficult enough after having lived through a deliberately instituted nuclear event (or Holocaust) without the extra effort required to reorientate and sustain optimism even if nature had provided some of the impulses to make this possible.

Knowles notes that the Holocaust and the atomic bombings of Hiroshima and Nagasaki stand out as the 'most monumental acts of war' in human history. These events are monumental because of the level of killing involved but especially because of the killing of massive numbers of innocent people, including children. In the case of the atomic bombs, a large, although like the human toll indeterminate, number of animals were also exterminated. Of the research related to resilience and disasters, studies of Holocaust survivors are prominent. Knowles observes that research on atomic bomb survivors is in limited supply but the available data on health outcomes when compared with that from studies of people who had survived the Holocaust reveals similarities. These similarities occur, using Knowles' expressions, in both those who are merely surviving and those who have adjusted to the point of thriving. Moreover, the notions of surviving and thriving are also found in both types of secondary victims.

In making the link between the emotional, behavioural, and cognitive performance of Holocaust and atomic bomb survivors drawn by Knowles refers to the findings of a study examining resilience amongst the former by social worker Roberta Greene (2002). Greene identifies two sets of performances amongst Holocaust survivors that typified resilience. These are: (1)

consciously deciding to go on living, to celebrate life, and to adopt a positive attitude towards themselves; (2) to look to the future not the past.

The mental health of the survivor's children also requires subtle comprehension. Signs of psychological suffering in the offspring of Holocaust survivors (that is, those born after the end of the Second World War) have been found to differ depending on, for example, the mental health status of their survivor parents, the gender of the parents (Holocaust survivor mothers are more influential are on the mental well-being of their offspring than fathers), and the quality of child-parent attachment. Where there is one survivor parent the gender of that parent also mattered, as did having both parents who had survived the Holocaust. There is some evidence that Holocaust survivor offspring can experience heightened anxiety when faced with traumatic situations indicated by increased levels of the stress hormone cortisol. That said, there is more evidence that overall, the suffering of Holocaust survivors did not seem to differ markedly from emotional distress and diagnoses of mental disorder than the offspring of non-survivors offspring (Dashorst *et al.*, 2019).

People who are diagnosed with severe forms of mental disorder, or if not diagnosed display signs of severe psychological suffering, may affect members of their family and others with whom or have close associations (Epstein, 1979). The expressed emotional, behavioural, and cognitive, psychopathological performances provide benchmarks for what may then be internalised and copied by significant others. This is particularly so with parent-child relationships diagnosed, for example, with anxiety, depression, or PTSD. It is unsurprising, therefore, that there is a group of Holocaust survivor offspring with higher-than-expected incidents of diagnosed mental disorders. This was, however, a small minority of the total number of survivor offspring (Dashorst *et al.*, 2019).

Natan Kellermann is a psychologist and psycho-dramatist. He is also a 'next generation' child of Holocaust survivors:

> At the age of fifteen, A-8816 arrived at Auschwitz-Birkenau with her family..in 1944.... [H]er parents and younger brothers and sisters were sent to the gas chambers....[B]arely alive, she was liberated by the British army in Bergen-Belson... [T]hereafter she gave birth to two boys, I was the second of the two.
>
> (Kellermann, 2009, p.vii)

Kellermann writes about how he has lived with gruesome images of the Holocaust throughout his life and absorbed the emotional burdens of his parents. But he is a champion for subtle academic and clinical analysis. The nuanced appreciation of the psychological harm to the next generation of the survivors of the concentration camp should include pinpointing and probing the characteristics of those families most are at risk of trauma transmission and the mechanisms through which transmission becomes possible. Furthermore, the offspring of the children of the survivors may need to be examined to assess if trauma transmission is persistent inter-generationally and is so then assistance offered. When psychological suffering does occur, there is no predictable single form or pattern to that suffering. There may be one type of emotional distress or a mixture of, for example, sadness, apprehension, and guilt. There may be substantial differences in the level of suffering endured from these negative emotions, and no assurance that suffering one is less likely to cause more suffering than suffering a mix. Moreover, what is given less attention, understandably, are the deleterious feelings of the surviving active participants in and passive observers of genocide, and the potential for trauma transmission in their offspring (Kellermann, 2009).

The focus on the psychological damage done to survivors of the Second World War concentration camps and the atrocities committed therein, and the effects of their offspring, is also to be expected. The horrific experiences of those who didn't survive and those who didn't still need to be, recognised, and remembered. Help of whatever hue offered to the now small number of survivors still alive and their children for as long as needed (Dashorst *et al.*, 2019). What is perhaps unexpected, and more so than many other disastrous events, is that most of the survivors displayed resilience not only to survive in the first place but to continue surviving once they left those camps. The aptitudes associated with both coping with the past and hoping for the future are as potent to pass on to offspring and have been more plentiful than psychopathological propensities. But another gradation in understanding any element of human performance concerns avoiding simplistic dichotomies such as, on the one side vulnerability to psychological suffering and diagnoses of mental disorder ensuing from trauma, and on the other an ability to cope psychologically (Kellermann, 2009).

A meta-analysis has been conducted by psychologist Efral Barel and her colleagues of the accumulative research from 1964 to 2008 on the long-term psychological and physical consequences of the Holocaust for survivors. The overall conclusion of the authors of this meta-analysis is equivocal. Efral Barel and her colleagues found that some of the research indicated that survivors had coped less well than comparative groups without involvement in the Holocaust. For example, they suffered substantially more from PTSD. However, other studies they examined also found that Holocaust survivors had not suffered significantly more from physical ill-health, anxiety, and cognitive dysfunction, and had shown 'remarkable resilience'. The authors of the meta-analysis suggest this ability to cope having survived the horrors of the concentration camps could be explained in part by the survivors employing what they refer to as 'defensive mechanisms' to prevent potential psychological disintegration and allow the shoring-up of their psychological stamina. One of these psychological shields mentioned by the authors is 'repression', that is the subconscious blocking of painful thoughts emanating from traumatic experiences. But another of these defensive mechanisms according to the authors was social. Those survivors of the Holocaust who moved to Israel compared to those who had moved to other countries seemed to have had better protection from the otherwise harmful psychological of their wartime experiences (Barel *et al.*, 2010).

Importantly, Barel and her colleagues point out that the emotional 'scars' of the Holocaust did not heal but they did not necessarily prevent personal growth and social adjustment. Most of the survivors of the Holocaust were children during the Second World War. In adulthood post-war they successfully built up their lives despite the extreme traumas they had undergone. They gained employment, got married, had children, and engaged in community commitments:

> Our investigation suggests that Holocaust survivors demonstrate remarkable resilience in adapting to their personal, social, and communal life.
>
> (Barel *et al.*, 2010, p.694)

There is a warning, however, from the authors of this study, that as the survivors enter old age their repressed memories, may surface. Retirement, ill-health, the loss of a partner, and loneliness, may activate reminiscence and in so doing furnish psychological instability.

The equivocation in the research, suggests Barel and her colleagues, may have arisen because of the adoption of different theoretical and methodological approaches. Some of the studies were dedicated to a psychoanalytical perspective (or it's the less analytically purist psychodynamic offshoot). From this perspective, an individual's childhood experiences are paramount in the development of the adult's performance, especially her/his personality, and mental well-being. Severe adversity in children will, from this perspective, lead to much and long-lasting distress unless tackled therapeutically. Non-psychodynamic approaches have been guided by more pragmatic research questions (that is, less constrained by preceding theoretical creeds), or are looking for evidence of positive outcomes such as functional adaptation as exemplified by coping performances and hopefulness.

This comprehensive and systematic review of research into the effects of the Holocaust on survivors reaped a vital insight that can provide lessons for the survivors of subsequent genocides. This insight is that contained within the body of knowledge relating to Holocaust survival is the core contradiction that while most if not all survivors to some degree suffer psychologically, and some of that suffering may lead to psychiatric classification, many if not most not only cope the consequences of their experiences but have fulfilling lives. Moreover, resilience and vulnerability co-exist both in the overall population of Holocaust survivors and among individual survivors.

But the view that social crises, perhaps those of the severe in their adverse impact while they are happening, can lead to beneficial changes for people and in society, can be challenged. The claim that war has positive spin-offs ignores the reality that war is a 'negative-sum activity' in terms of the loss of life and social destruction. The latter includes the denting of some and the wrecking of other moral, ethical, and legal codes, and the ruining economies as well (perhaps the not-so-unfortunate) ruination of established and aspir-ant empires, long-standing monarchies and autocracies. A saner path to soci-etal progress could have been in the offing without the journey having to be littered with material debris, dead bodies, and damaged minds (Broadberry and Harrison, 2005).

Antibiotics and Antipsychotics

There is not the possibility of running experiments to test whether any posi-tive outcomes of negative events on the scale of a world war could compare with the devastation associated with such events. Although it is problematic to separate catastrophe from fortuity, human progress and the development of sophisticated civilisations are stimulated as much by a combination of serendipity, speculation, sagacity, and commercialism, as they are by social crisis resulting from contagions and conflicts, or a mixture of all of these the factors.

For example, the discovery of antibiotics can be connected to antecedent social crises such as the high levels of morbidity and mortality from wide-spread diseases including pneumonia, syphilis, gonorrhoea, and diarrheal infections amongst the two world war combatants as well as civilians. It was also the upshot of thousands of was built on thousands of years of phil-osophical musing and rudimentary scientific theorising and trialling – and good fortune. One of the most significant progressions in medical knowledge came about in 1928 when Alexander Fleming, physician and microbiologist at St. Mary's Hospital in London, had a 'eureka' moment (Brown, 2005). He happened to notice that the fungus *Penicillium notatum* (later renamed *Penicillium chrysogenum*) had contaminated a culture plate of Staphylococ-cus bacteria he had unintentionally left uncovered.

Ancient civilisations used a variety of natural ingredients (for example, herbs and honey) in their attempts to fight infections (Gould, 2016). Some more-modern antibiotics may have been available in ancient times Traces of the antibiotic tetracyclines have been found in human skeletons in Nubia (an area along the river Nile) dating from when the Romans occupied Egypt. Throughout the century before Fleming's providential finding, the inhibition of bacterial pathogenic growth when in contact with other microbes (as well as toxic chemicals such as arsenic) had been noticed by physicians and scien-tists. Experiments using moulds that were part of the penicillin genus had also been conducted with promising results, but their elemental properties had not been understood and their potential had not been unexploited. Fleming, on the other hand, was dogged in his desire to see his discovery go mainstream.

Following this fortuitous finding by Fleming, al-be-it abetted by a long history of preceding minor eureka moments and major historical events, there was another combination of personal and societal factors that enabled the benefits of antibiotics to be realised by (eventually) the world's population. It wasn't just that antibiotics readjusted the balance in the conflict between infectious (bacterial) diseases and humans in favour of the latter. The invention of these drugs and their application as prophylactics meant that the chance of post-surgery infection was reduced greatly, hereby allowing more protracted operations could be undertaken and complicated techniques, could be employed. Moreover, are used regularly to fight secondary bacterial infections from diseases caused by viruses.

The curing of debilitating and deadly diseases globally stemmed from the effective production and distribution of these 'wonder drugs' by profit-making pharmaceutical companies and initially with the assistance and insistence of governments. It is a mixture of similar factors, including bad fortune, that antimicrobial resistance caused in the main by the hyper-consumption of antibiotics now furnish a serious social crisis that threatens the lives of millions of people and possibly transporting medical knowledge and human health back to the dark ages (Bowater, 2016). Many present antibiotics are failing to cure past diseases and with few prospective replacements with the potency to tackle microbial 'superbugs', further bacterial pandemics, possibly caused by vulnerability to further viral pandemics, will increase the threat to the survival of humanity if concurrent with the climate emergency and the concomitant undermining of animal life and the viability of soil for growing crops, and thereby jeopardising food security. The COVID-19 pandemic provides a paragon of the paradox regarding antibiotics. They are both wonderful and worrisome inventions. Both their unnecessary and appropriate use in patients who have been affected severely by the COVID-19 virus may have contributed to the problem of antimicrobial resistance (Chen et al., 2023).

The story of antipsychotic medication offers another example of how there are many aspects to apparent personal and societal advancement. Antipsychotic drug development followed a lengthy and torturous course, replete with chance and ambiguous empirical findings, and power struggles among those who wanted to reap what seemed to be the therapeutic and commercial rewards of using this novel method of physical treatment (Shen, 1999). Chemical combinations for what was to become reformulated to perform as antipsychotic drugs had been designed as far back as 1891 as antimalarials, for the control of allergies, and in surgical procedures for their anaesthetic effect. Since these original antipsychotics became used (and overused) in the early 1950s, there have been further chemical concoctions designed to perform in similar ways to the original wave of antipsychotics but without their serious side-effects. The notion that these drugs offered a solution to psychosis was swallowed wholeheartedly by the majority of Western psychiatrists, and contemporary psychiatry throughout most of the world relies mainly on these and other pharmaceuticals for the treatment of most diagnosed mental disorders (Morrall, 2017).

The societal context for this adherence to a form of treatment that seemed to offer the miraculous remedy for otherwise intractable and incapacitating mental disorders was the existence of a multiplicity of liberating movements occurring after the Second World War. The general shift towards a freer and fairer society, along with accumulating reports from journalists and sociologists about the mistreatment of mental hospital patients and the growing cost of maintaining these ageing facilities meant that it was no longer tenable to keep legions of people hidden away from the rest of society (Miller and Rose, 1986).

But, as with antibiotics and many other supposed elements of progress in the human condition and societal sophistication, the use of drugs of this sort and pharmaceutics *per se* to deal with psychological suffering is considered a bad fortune. Despite billions of these drugs having been prescribed, they are at best palliative not curative, and bestow severe side-effects. Furthermore, they affirm the power of psychiatry and medicalisation of psychological suffering and also assist the spread of mental-healthism. As mentioned above, psychiatric power and psychological suffering are highly contestable approaches to psychological suffering, and mental-healthism has several undesirable repercussions.

Just as the law of unexpected consequences applies to social crises, the law of unintended consequences applies to medical interventions, especially drugs. Efficaciousness of medical pharmaceuticals coexists with short-term side-effects, long-term sequelae, feebleness, uselessness, incongruousness, and the unintended impediment or intended benefit of the placebo effect.

Medical intervention has now stretched beyond body and mind. Medical practitioners can now write 'social' prescriptions. Social prescribing creates a formal way for primary care services to refer patients to a variety of non-clinical services (Evans, 2021). The establishment of social prescribing as a medical intervention is aimed at tackling specific forms of psychological suffering such as loneliness. The lack of connection between this medical intervention and the individual's social context has been recognised. To address this omission new variants of social prescribing are proposed. One variant, 'Community-enhanced Social Prescribing', is intended to integrate medically prescribed individual activities (for example, gardening, dancing, and walking) with community activity. The advocates of this variant proclaim that it has the potential to improve the well-being of both individuals and the community (Morris *et al.*, 2022).

However, the 'social' part of social prescribing is misleading no matter that some models advocate increasing the connection between personal performance and communal set-ups. Loneliness, while it is experienced as a personal problem and one that could lead to medical intervention and a possible diagnosis of mental disorder is associated with, for example, depression and/or anxiety, is a social disorder. The more accurate term for loneliness is 'social isolation' in terms of its causes and consequences. Social disorders cannot be cured by medical prescription even if these supposed remedies contain extra community ingredients. Social disorders require the remedying of society, not the sufferer, and not the palliative and perfunctory medical measure of 'social prescribing'. Indeed, social prescribing camouflages the actual origins of social isolation thereby avoiding the proper prescription of societal variation.

Factual Hopefulness

Hans Rosling a Swedish physician, a scholar on international health, argues for more 'factfulness'. For Rosling (2018) there are facts that support hopefulness. Rosling argues that the world with or without a social crisis is saner than usually suggested is a fact. 'Factfluness' for Rosling is the stress-reducing habit of only carrying opinions for which you have strong supporting facts. Rosling suggests that what stops people from relying on facts is that frequently they that they don't know what they don't know, and even best guesses are informed by unconscious and predictable biases. It turns out that the world, claims Rosling, for all its imperfections, is in a much better state than is usually believed by the public and purported by the media.

Rosling accepts, however, that the world does face genuine problems some of which are formidable, such as wars, natural disasters, the climate emergency, and inequality. He was writing prior to the COVID-19 pandemic. But he argues that year by year, the world is improving. Notable improvements have been in life expectancy which has more than doubled in the last two centuries, the proportion of people living in extreme poverty has almost halved, and the number of fatalities from conflict has been falling since the Second World War although there are blips in this trend (he gives the examples of fatalities for the Syrian civil war, and terrorism). Rosling refers to the slow and silent 'miracle of human progress', so slow and silent that it doesn't make for media headlines where new conflict or contagion does.

Summary

Human kindness and cooperativeness are crucial for the survival of kinship genes and for the procreation and endurance of the species. This is the 'selfish' side of human nature. However, plenty of species are, as far as can be ascertained, sustained without such qualities. Humans, however, exist and persist because they have formed sophisticated cultures. There is a 'selfless' side to human nurturing. But both the nature and nurture sides have inconsistencies. The physiological make-up of humans is sensitive to unselfishness and selfishness intrudes on some societal set-ups. Nevertheless, the overall impact of human nature and nurturing is to craft and coset kindness and cooperativeness, with regular heroics added to the mix of prosocial performances and mutuality.

As in 'normal' times (that is when there aren't any discernible and widespread social crises) social schisms exist alongside societal solidarities. Communities can solidify through kindness and cooperation in times of social crisis but are susceptible to dissolution when social stability seems *in situ* but severe social schisms persist.

Sociologist Mary Holmes (2016) wants a more her discipline to be more hopeful. She argues for sociology to have a more optimistic view of the world. There is for Holmes too much focus on the world's problems to the point whereby sociology seems to have pathologised much of social life. Pessimism for Holmes limits the sociological imagination.

These signs of sanity, kindness and cooperation, social solidarity, and coping and coping, do not displace the societal insanities of violence, inequality, insecurity, selfishness, and stupidity. But they do all allow a future sane society with far less psychological suffering to be imagined.

Notes

1 United Nations Children's Fund was originally called the United Nations International Children's Emergency Fund and used the acronym 'UNICEF'. The acronym has been retained.
2 There are two 'Ward's mentioned in the book. Therefore I have written each name in full.

References

Abrams Z (2021) The Case for Kindness. American Psychological Association, August. https://www.apa.org/news/apa/kindness-mental-health [accessed 15th March, 2023]

Al Jazeera (2023) Major Earthquakes Hit Turkey, Syria: Who Is Stepping up to Help? https://www.aljazeera.com/news/2023/2/6/major-earthquake-hits-turkey-syria-which-countries-offered-help [accessed 7th February, 2023]

Alberti F (2020) Coronavirus Is Revitalising the Concept of Community for the 21st Century. The Conversation, 29th April. https://theconversation.com/coronavirus-is-revitalising-the-concept-of-community-for-the-21st-century-135750 [accessed 7th May, 2020]

Alexander P, Berri A, Moran D, Reay D and Rounsevell M (2020) The Global Environmental Paw Print of Pet Food. *Global Environmental Change*, November, 65(102153). https://www.sciencedirect.com/science/article/pii/S0959378020307366 [accessed 17th March, 2023]

AlphaFold Team (2020) AlphaFold: A Solution to a 50-year-old Grand Challenge in Biology. DeepMind, 30 November. https://deepmind.com/blog/article/alphafold-a-solution-to-a-50-year-old-grand-challenge-in-biology [accessed 2nd December, 2020]

Andrés O (2022) COVID May Have Made Us Less Materialistic – New Research. The Conversation, 17th February. https://theconversation.com/covid-may-have-made-us-less-materialistic-new-research-175890 [accessed 19th February, 2022]

Barel E, IJzendoorn M, Sagi-Schwartz A and Bakermans-Kranenburg M (2010) Surviving the Holocaust: A Meta-analysis of the Long-term Sequelae of a Genocide. *Psychological Bulletin*, 136(5), pp.677–698.

BBC News (2023) Covid Origin: Why the Wuhan Lab-leak Theory Is So Disputed, 1st March. https://www.bbc.co.uk/news/world-asia-china-57268111 [accessed 26th March, 2023]

Borkowska M and Laurence J (2021) Coming Together or Coming Apart? Changes in Social Cohesion During the Covid-19 Pandemic in England. *European Societies*, 23[supplement 1], pp.1–19.

Born This Way Foundation (2023) #BeKind21. https://bornthisway.foundation/current-programs/bekind21/ [accessed 16th March, 2023]

Bowater S (2016) *The Microbes Fight Back: Antibiotic Resistance*. London: Royal Society of Chemistry.

Broadberry S and Harrison M (2005) (editors) *The Economics and World War 1*. Cambridge: Cambridge University Press.

Brown K (2005) *Penicillin Man: Alexander Fleming and the Antibiotic Revolution*. Cheltenham: The History Press.

Brueggemann A *et al.* [100> co-authors] (2021) Changes in the Incidence of Invasive Disease due to Streptococcus Pneumoniae, Haemophilus Influenzae, and Neisseria Meningitidis during the COVID-19 Pandemic in 26 Countries and Territories in the Invasive Respiratory Infection Surveillance Initiative: A Prospective Analysis of Surveillance Data. *The Lancet*, 3(6), E360–E370. https://www.thelancet.com/journals/landig/article/PIIS2589-7500(21)00077-7/fulltext [accessed 13th December, 2021].

Captain Tom Foundation (2023) *The Captain Tom Foundation: Sharing Stories of Hope*. https://captaintom.org/story-1 [accessed 21st March, 2023]

Centers for Disease Control and Prevention (2022) Diseases That Can Spread Between Animals and People. https://www.cdc.gov/healthypets/diseases/index.html [accessed 13th March 2023]

Chen J, Hoang H, Yaskina M, Kabbani D, Doucette K, Smith S, Lau C, Stewart J, Remtulla S, Zurek K, Schultz M, Koriyama-McKenzie H and Cervera C (2023) Efficacy and Safety of Antimicrobial Stewardship Prospective Audit and Feedback in Patients Hospitalised with COVID-19. *The Lancet*, 23rd January. https://www.thelancet.com/journals/laninf/article/PIIS1473-3099(22)00832-5/fulltext [accessed 8th February, 2023]

Cohn S (2018) *Epidemics: Hate and Compassion from the Plague of Athens to AIDS*. Oxford: Oxford University Press.

Coulter L (2020) Coronavirus Shows we Must Get Serious about the Well-Being of Animals. The Conversation, 24th May. https://theconversation.com/coronavirus-shows-we-must-get-serious-about-the-well-being-of-animals-138872 [accessed 24th August, 2021]

Darley J and Latané B (1968) Bystander Intervention in Emergencies: Diffusion of Responsibility. *Journal of Personality and Social Psychology*, 8(4), pp.377–383.

Dashorst P, Mooren T, Kleber R, Jong P and Huntjens R (2019) Intergenerational Consequences of the Holocaust on Offspring Mental Health: A Systematic Review of Associated Factors and Mechanisms. *European Journal of Psychotraumatology*, 10(1), 1654065. https://www.tandfonline.com/doi/pdf/10.1080/20008198.2019.1654065 [accessed 30th January, 2023]

Deckers L (2014) (4th edition) *Motivation: Biological, Psychological, and Environmental*. Boston, MA: Allyn & Bacon.

Dineen K (2020) Why Resilience Isn't Always the Answer to Coping with Challenging Times. The Conversation, 29th September. https://theconversation.com/why-resilience-isnt-always-the-answer-to-coping-with-challenging-times-145796. [accessed 30th November, 2020]

Durkheim E (1895) *Les Règles de la Méthode Sociologique*. Paris: Alcan.

Epstein H (1979) *Children of the Holocaust: Conversations with Sons and Daughters of the Survivors*. New York: Putnam and Sons.

Erdem S (2022) A Need for Earthquake Diplomacy. *The New European*, 11th November. https://www.theneweuropean.co.uk/a-need-for-earthquake-diplomacy/ [accessed 10th January, 2023]Etzioni A (2014) Communitarianism Revisited. *Journal of Political Ideologies*, 19(3), pp.241–260.

Evans C (2021) Covid: Loneliness a 'Bigger Health Risk Than Smoking or Obesity'. BBC News, 27th June. https://www.bbc.co.uk/news/uk-wales-57622710 [accessed 28th June, 2021]Fancourt D, Steptoe A and Bradbury A (2022) Tracking the Psychological and Social Consequences of the COVID-19 Pandemic across the UK Population: Findings, Impact, and Recommendations from the COVID-19 Social Study (March 2020 – April 2022). London: University College London.

Fonseca C, Pettitt J, Woollard A, Rutherford A, Bickmore W, Ferguson-Smith A and Hurst L (2023) People with More Extreme Attitudes Towards Science Have Self-Confidence in Their Understanding of Science, Even If This Is Not Justified. *PLoS Biology*, 21(1), [e3001915]. https://journals.plos.org/plosbiology/article?id=10.1371/journal.pbio.3001915 [accessed 27th April, 2023]

Franco Z and Zimbardo P (2016) The Banality of Heroism. Greater Good, 1st September. https://greatergood.berkeley.edu/article/item/the_banality_of_heroism [accessed 23rd March, 2023]

Friedlingstein P *et al.* [approx. 80 co-authors] (2020) Global Carbon Budget 2020. *Earth Systems Science Data*, 12(4), pp.3269–3340.

Fritz C (1996 original 1961) *Disasters and Mental Health: Therapeutic Principles Drawn from Disaster Studies*. Newark, DE: University of Delaware. https://udspace.udel.edu/bitstream/handle/19716/1325/HC%2010.pdf?sequence=1&isAllowed=y [accessed 22nd September, 2020].

Gilbert S and Green C (2022) *Vaxxers: The Inside Story of the Oxford AstraZeneca Vaccine and the Race Against the Virus*. London: Hodder and Stoughton.

Goldacre B (2009) *Bad Science*. London: Harper.

Goldacre B (2012) *Bad Pharma: How Drug Companies Mislead Doctors and Harm Patients*. London: Fourth Estate.

Goldacre B (2014) *I Think You'll Find It's a Bit More Complicated Than That*. London: Fourth Estate.

Goldin I (2021) *Rescue: From Global Crisis to a Better World*. London: Hodder & Stoughton.

Goldman E and Galea S (2014) Mental Health Consequences of Disasters. *Annual Review of public Health*, 35, pp.169–183.

Greene R. (2002) Holocaust Survivors: A Study in Resilience. *Journal of Gerontological Social Work*, 37(1), pp.3–18.Halpern D (2013) *Mental Health and the Built Environment: More Than Bricks and Mortar?* London: Routledge.

Hammond C (2022) *The Keys to Kindness: How to Be Kinder to Yourself, Others and the World*. Edinburgh: Canongate.

Harari Y (2017) *Homo Deus: A Brief History of Tomorrow*. London: Vintage.

Heneage J (2022) *The Shortest History of Greece*. Exeter: Old Street.

Holmes M (2016) *Sociology for Optimists*. London: Sage.

Holz N and Lowery T (2022) 9 Acts of Kindness Towards Ukraine's People That Will Give You Hope. Global Citizen, 3rd March. https://www.globalcitizen.org/en/content/dinge-die-uns-gerade-hoffnung-machen/ [accessed 23rd March, 2023]

Jacob B, Mawson A, Payton M and Guignard J (2008) Disaster Mythology and

Fact: Hurricane Katrina and Social Attachment. *Public Health Reports*, 123(5), pp.555–566.

Johnson B (2021) Captain Sir Tom Moore: Boris Johnson Pays Tribute. BBC News [video clip], 2nd February. https://www.bbc.co.uk/news/av/uk-55911044 [accessed 23rd March, 2023]

Kavedžija I (2022) Wellbeing: How Living Well Together Works for the Common Good. The Conversation, 16th February. https://theconversation.com/wellbeing-how-living-well-together-works-for-the-common-good-176722 [accessed 19th February, 2022]Kellermann N (2009) *Holocaust Trauma: Psychological Effects and Treatment*. New York: iUniverse Inc.

Kelman L (2020) Disaster By Choice: How Our Actions Turn Natural Hazards Into Catastrophes. Oxford, UK: Oxford University Press.

Kelman L (2021) 'Natural' Disasters Are Due To Societal Failures – So, Here's a Six-Point Pandemic Recovery Plan. The Conversation, 21st June. https://theconversation.com/natural-disasters-are-due-to-societal-failures-so-heres-a-six-point-pandemic-recovery-plan-161719 [accessed 18th April, 2022]

Kesternich I, Siflinger B, Smith J and Winter J (2014) The Effects of World War II on Economic and Health Outcomes Across Europe. *The Review of Economics and Statistics*, 96(1), pp.103–118.Knowles A (2011) Resilience Among Japanese Atomic Bomb Survivors. *International Nursing Review*, 58(1), pp.54–60.

Kobayashi T, Maeda M, Nakayama C, Takebayashi Y, Sato H, Setou N, Momoi M, Horikoshi N, S Yasumura and Ohto H (2022) Disaster Resilience Reduces Radiation-Related Anxiety Among Affected People 10 Years After the Fukushima Daiichi Nuclear Power Plant Accident. Frontiers in Public Health, 14th. July, 10(839442) https://www.frontiersin.org/articles/10.3389/fpubh.2022.839442/full [accessed 3rd August, 2023]

Legal and General (2020) *The Isolation Economy Report*. London: Legal and General.

Litman T (2021) *Urban Sanity: Understanding Urban Mental Health Impacts and How to Create Saner, Happier Cities*. Victoria: Transport Policy Institute.

Litman T (2022) *New Mobilities: Smart Planning for Emerging Transportation Technologies*. Washington, DC: Island Press.

Longmuir C and Agyapon (2022) Social and Mental Health Impact of Nuclear Disaster in Survivors: A Narrative Review. Behavioral Sciences, 11(8): 113. https://www.ncbi.nlm.nih.gov/pmc/articles/PMC8389263/ [accessed 26th January, 2023]

MacCurdy J (1943) *The Structure of Morale*. Cambridge, UK: Cambridge University Press.

Makwana N (2019) Disaster and its Impact on Mental Health: A Narrative Review. *Journal of Family Medicine and Primary Care*, 8(10), pp.3090–3095.

Manning R, Levine M and Collins A (2007) The Kitty Genovese Murder and the Social Psychology of Helping: The Parable of the 38 Witnesses. *American Psychologist*, 62(6), pp.555–562.

Margana L, Bhogal M, Bartlett J and Farrelly D (2019) The Roles of Altruism, Heroism, and Physical Attractiveness in Female Mate Choice. *Personality and Individual Differences*, 137(15), pp.126–130.

McCay L and Litman T (2021) *Centre for Urban Design and Mental Health: Facts and Figures*. Centre for Urban Design and Mental Health. https://www.urbandesign-mentalhealth.com/facts-and-figures.html [accessed 17th August, 2021]

McCay L and Roe J (2021) Covid Has Shown Us That Our Neighbourhood Could Be Harming Our Health. The Independent, 14th August. https://www.independent.co.uk/voices/cities-health-impact-wellbeing-pandemic-b1899986.html   [accessed 17th August, 2021].

McKie R (2020) The Vaccine Miracle: How Scientists Waged the Battle Against Covid-19. The Observer, 6th December.

Mental Health Foundation (2022a) How Can a Pet Help My Mental Health? https://www.mentalhealth.org.uk/explore-mental-health/a-z-topics/pets-and-mental-health [accessed 16th March, 2023]

Mental Health Foundation (2022b) What Are the Health Benefits of Altruism? *Mental Health Foundation*. https://www.mentalhealth.org.uk/explore-mental-health/articles/what-are-health-benefits-altruism [accessed 23rd August, 2022]

Meulen R (2017) *Solidarity and Justice in Health and Social Care*. Cambridge: Cambridge University Press.

Milgram S (1974) *Obedience to Authority: An Experimental View*. New York: Harper and Row.

Miller P and Rose N (1986) *The Power of Psychiatry*. Cambridge: Polity.

Modgil R (2021) Actions, Even Small Ones, Can Force Change [when the world seems overwhelming]. i news, 28th August.

Moore T (2020) *Tomorrow Will Be a Good Day: My Autobiography*. London: Penguin Michael Joseph.

Moore T (2021) *Captain Tom's Life Lessons: Above All Be Kind*. London: Penguin Michael Joseph.

Morrall P (2009) *Sociology and Health: An Introduction*. London: Routledge.

Morrall P (2017) *Madness: Ideas about Insanity*. Abingdon, UK: Routledge.

Morris D, Thomas P, Ridley J and Webber M (2022) Community-Enhanced Social Prescribing: Integrating Community in Policy and Practice. *International Journal of Community Wellbeing*, 5(1), pp.179–195.Nelson-Coffey S, Fritz M, Lyubomirsky S, and Cole S (2017) Kindness in the Blood: A Randomized Controlled Trial of the Gene Regulatory Impact of Prosocial Behavior. *Psychoneuroendocrinology*, 81(July), pp.8–13.

Nieuwerburgh C and Nacif A (2020) COVID Vaccines Will Be Here Soon – In the Meantime, Here's How to Stay Resilient. The Conversation, 27th November. https://theconversation.com/covid-vaccines-will-be-here-soon-in-the-meantime-heres-how-to-stay-resilient-151000 [accessed 30th November, 2020].

Official Website of Ukraine (2023) Defenders of Freedom. https://war.ukraine.ua/heroes/

Passerini E (2000) Disasters as Agents of Social Change in Recovery and Reconstruction. *Natural Hazards Review*, 1(2), pp.67–72.

Pinker S (2011) *The Better Angels of Our Nature: Why Violence Has Declined*. New York: Viking, New York NY.

Post S (2005) Altruism, Happiness, and Health: It's Good to Be Good. *International Journal of Behavioral Medicine*, 12(2), pp.66–77.

Post S (2009) It's Good to Be Good: Science Says It's So. Research Demonstrates that People Who Help Others Usually Have Healthier, Happier Lives. *Health Progress*, 90(4), pp.18–25.

Putin V (2023) Congratulations on the Occasion of Defender of the Fatherland Day. http://en.kremlin.ru/events/president/news/70575 [accessed 23rd March, 2023]

Rahman A, Naslund J, Betancourt T, Black C, Bhan A, Byansi W, Chen H, Gaynes B, Restrepo C, Gouveia L, Hamdani S, Marsch L, Petersen I, Bahar O, Shields-Zeeman L, Ssewamala F and Wainberg M (2020) The NIMH Global Mental Health Research Community and COVID-19. *The Lancet*, 7(10), pp.384–386.

Roe J and McCay L (2021) *Restorative Cities: Urban Design for Mental Health and Wellbeing*. London: Bloomsbury.

Rutherford A and Fry H (2021) *Rutherford & Fry's Complete Guide to Absolutely Everything*. London: Bantum.

Saladié O, Bustamante E and Gutiérrez A (2020) COVID-19 Lockdown and Reduction of Traffic Accidents in Tarragona Province, Spain. *Transportation Research Interdisciplinary Perspectives*, 8(100218), November. https://www.sciencedirect.com/science/article/pii/S2590198220301299 [accessed 13th December, 2020]

Sandhu S (2021) How to Be Inspired By Failure (and Come Back Better). The i Newspaper, 1st July.

Scott A and Goethals G (2010) *Heroes: What They Do and Why We Need Them*. New York: Oxford University Press.

Shen W (1999) A History of Antipsychotic Drug Development. *Comprehensive Psychiatry*, 40(60, pp.407-414.

Sitrin M and *Colectiva Semrara* (2020) (editors) *Pandemic Solidarity: Mutual Aid During the Covid-19 Crisi*. London: Pluto.

Slack P (1988) Responses to Plague in Early Modern Europe: The Implications of Public Health. *Social Research*, 55(3), pp.433–453.

Southwick S, Bonanno G, Masten A, Panter-Brick C and Yehuda R (2014) Resilience Definitions, Theory, and Challenges: Interdisciplinary Perspectives. *European Journal of Psychotraumatology*, 5(1), p.25338. https://www.tandfonline.com/doi/full/10.3402/ejpt.v5.25338 [accessed 3rd January, 2022]

Spinney L (2017) *Pale Rider: The Spanish Flu of 1918 and How It Changed the World*. London: Vintage.

Szalavitz M (2012) How Disasters Bring Out Our Kindness. TimeHealth, 31st October. https://healthland.time.com/2012/10/31/how-disasters-bring-out-our-kindness/ [accessed 3rd December, 2021]

United Nations Children's Fund (2022a) Called to Serve. New York: United Nations Children's Fund. https://www.unicef.org/uganda/stories/called-serve [accessed 21st March, 2023]

United Nations Children's Fund (2022b) The Unsung Pandemic Heroes. New York: United Nations Children's Fund. https://www.unicef.org/coronavirus/unsung-heroes-pandemic [accessed 21st March, 2023]

University of Sussex (2023) The Kindness Test. https://www.sussex.ac.uk/research/centres/kindness/research/thekindnesstest [accessed 15th March, 2023]

Vella S and Pai N (2019) A Theoretical Review of Psychological Resilience: Defining Resilience and Resilience Research over the Decades. *Archive of Medicine & Health Science*, 7(2), pp.233–239.

Ward M (2020) How the Modern World Was Shaped by Epidemics 500 Years Ago. The Conversation, September 18th. https://theconversation.com/how-the-modern-world-was-shaped-by-epidemics-500-years-ago-145905 [accessed 29th September, 2020]

Ward, M (2022) CoronaDiaries: Documenting the everyday lived experiences of a global pandemic. Digital Humanties Lab, Swansea University. https://collections.

swansea.ac.uk/s/coronadiaries/page/home [accessed 18th October, 2022]Wilde L (2013) *Global Solidarity*. Edinburgh, UK: Edinburgh University Press.

Wilks Y (2019) *Artificial Intelligence: Modern Magic or Dangerous Future?* London: Icon.

Zimbardo P, Haney C, Banks W and Jaffe D. (1973) The Mind is a Formidable Jailer: A Pirandellian Prison. New York Times Magazine, 8th April, section 6, p.36.

Zinoviev A (1986) *Homo Sovieticus*. New York: Grove Atlantic.

Conclusion

In the introduction, I outlined the idea for this book and its aims. The idea was to progress from perceiving society as mainly a repository of entrenched cultural and structural 'insanities' as identified in my previous book titled *Insane Society: A Sociology of Mental Health* (Morrall, 2020). That these societal insanities (inequality; violence; selfishness; insecurity; and stupidity) are primary producers of psychological suffering along with suffering physically is not surprising. Nor is it surprising that at times these insanities either singularly or collaboratively, when they become extreme, can cause a social crisis. The societal insanities of violence, inequality, selfishness insecurity, and stupidity are reified when human lifestyles create the conditions for pandemics and epidemics, engage in warfare, and destroy their habitat to such an extent that it risks destroying life on earth. In turn, social crises are generally considered responsible for generating further suffering.

But in this book, I have presented if not an alternative perspective on how people and society fare even when faced with catastrophic contagions and conflicts, then a much more positive perspective. The insanities haven't disappeared but at least they partly dissipate amongst signs of societal sanity such as kindness, cooperation, solidarity, coping, and hoping. Furthermore, what has been emphasised in this book is that society's sanities directly and substantially affect mental health, in a beneficial way. Notwithstanding lethal diseases, terrible cruelties, the destruction of physical environments, collapsing of communities, the pervasiveness of mendacity, ignorance, and the apparent ubiquity of despair and disempowerment, people do good and sensible things as do some social institutions, and personal and societal goodness and sense is good and sensible for mental health.

Signs of sanity are not just the celebrated and superlative deeds of magnanimity, philanthropy, comparison, altruism, unanimity, science, or politics. There are the multitudinous, mundane, and minuscule endeavours that seed those venerated successes and the isolated and inconspicuous acts that fertilise the foundations for a saner society and thereby of psychological solidity.

However, society and humans are imbued with complications and contradictions. Indeed, one such complicated contradiction arises from how social

DOI: 10.4324/9781003223757-6

crises seem to affect both society and mental health both negatively and positively. Contagions and conflicts comprise the complexity and contradiction of calamity and consolation. Mental health and society, however, are interlinked no matter if society is in a crisis or not.

The issue of a purported mental health crisis has also been examined in the book, and an alternative viewpoint has been offered. This alternative viewpoint is that of 'mental-healthism'. 'Mental-healthism' is a concept that describes levels of psychological suffering as not in crisis in terms of levels of psychological suffering that may require professional input. If there is a crisis then it is one of a cultural shift whereby claims of psychological suffering (usually expressed as having a 'mental health problem') have become normalised. Most people, most of the time, when not encumbered with societal pressures to be otherwise, cope with most situations – including social crises.

Moreover, most of those coping do not lose hope for either a return to non-crisis normality or a better future.

On the theme of a better future, galvanising the personal, interpersonal, and communal positives from social crises can help make society less insane and psychological suffering subside. The signs of sanity seen in social crises may not solve all of society's insanities nor be the solution to all psychological suffering (humans and society are after all far too complex and contradictory for such a neat solution). But they do offer hope for a saner way of living and being.

Social crises lead to social change. The more catastrophic the crisis, the more considerable the change. The two world wars, the Black Death, and the global influenza epidemic were dramatic both in terms of their lethal effect on people and how they reshaped society. The long-lasting negative effects of COVID-19 are yet to be realised. The positive aspects of that pandemic are yet to be reified if they are at all but a new social contract to deal with ongoing and prospective crises and concomitant inequities has been called for by the United Nations, local and international trade unions, and nongovernmental organisations (Frey *et al.*, 2021).

Ian Goldin (2021) globalisation and development specialist, asks where the big thinkers are of today, the political and economic theorists who can rescue society from its insanities? Journalist Matthew Syed (2019) argues for the power of 'rebel ideas' and 'diverse thinking'. Enigmatic, eccentric, aberrant, weird, maverick, or controversial ideas must be heard and if not adopted at least adapted. Cognitive diversity can crack complexity, argues Syed.

Preparing and implementing a saner society could come about through one of three routes. The first is the ideological 'messiah' option. That is, await an individual who is inculcated with the right quality and quantity of intellectual and innovatory fervour (another Adam Smith, Karl Marx, or Amitai Etzioni) to formulate the foundations for a new 'sane' social contract. The second route is the anticipation that there will be an 'evolutionary' progressive unfolding of society from its insane state to a saner – perhaps even sane – state. From this viewpoint, humanity has evolved over millennia from a brutish existence in isolated and small units of hunters and gatherers, to belonging to a sophistically, safer, and more civilised and global society. The third route is the fusion of the first two, a combination of the otherwise incompatible notions that individuals make historical change possible and individuals who ostensibly are the catalysts for historical change are fashioned from their social situation.

There is yet another possibility, complete catastrophe. The accumulation and unresolving of social crises, including those arising from pandemics, nuclear warfare or accidents, and ecological disasters, could cause the near-complete collapse of life on Earth. From the ruins, life of one sort or another could either return to brutishness, replenish former forms of insanity or foment or fall-upon an inimitable mode of managing its existence. This fourth route to social change might be inevitable but is not advisable. The consequences of catastrophe, as has been witnessed at times of world wars and bloody revolutions, large-scale episodes of debilitating and deadly disease, and mass extinctions, may in the long-term lead to the resurgence of organic and/or inorganic life.

Possibly, social crises may have to mutate into mega catastrophes equivalent to the demise of the Aztec and Inca civilisations due mainly to disease-carrying invaders (Snowden, 2020; Williams, 2011), or the extra-terrestrial incursion that resulted in the extinction of three-quarters of the animal and plant species (Alvarez *et al.*, 1980).

However, the time needed for the regeneration may be extensive. In the case of the meteoric demise of much of plant life and many animal species, including the dinosaurs, replacement and diversification took millions of years (Lowery and Fraass, 2019). Moreover, the cost in terms of the suffering of sentient beings can also be catastrophic. Humans may cope with 'normal' social crises without the collapse of their individual or collective psyche but not with a colossal collapse of their social and physical environment.

Most societies most of the time are the upshot of 'adaptation' in the evolutionary sense. This is not to indulge the anthropomorphising, simplistic, and ethological reductionism of socio-biology or the teleological speculations and empirical flakiness of evolutionary psychology. However, just as genes and minds (whether the mind is considered separate from or conferred by a biological locale) are susceptible to maladaptation, so can society. Contagions and conflicts exemplify contemporary society's dysfunctional mutations. These deleterious deviations are jeopardising the survival not just of individuals, communities, and wider societal configurations, but the whole of the earth's ecosystem and thereby all of its biotic and abiotic components. Furthermore, it is highly unlikely that human life can persist on another planet (Saplakoglu, 2019). There must therefore be a very different way of thinking about how on earth organic and inorganic matter can survive.

Then there is the alleged threat from yet more of humanity's creations, 'Big Data' and Artificial Intelligence. Apart from the prospect of an advance in human society far more revolutionary than either that of the rise of industry and computer technology, the compiling of Big Data and its (mis)use by governments and corporations and the fast pace of developments in Artificial Intelligence is purported to threaten human autonomy (Clegg, 2017; Yudkowsky, 2023).

Political theorist Lawrence Wilde (2013) argues for political action towards global solidarity. He defines solidarity as a feeling of sympathy shared by people within and between groups that engenders mutual support and social inclusion. For Wilde 'radical humanism' is an ethical answer to the lack of social solidarity. Radical humanism, according to Wilde, promotes the ideas of shared humanity, rationality, compassion, cooperation, and productiveness. The latter Wilde uses in the sense meant by social-psychologist, psychoanalyst, philosopher, humanist, and sociologist Erich Fromm. Social sanity can be restored, Fromm (1955) suggests, by curtailing acquisitiveness, encouraging human compassion, comradeship, compromise, empathy, and love, and involvement in edifying and in the main shared activities such as art, music, and meaningful mental or physical work. Monbiot's ideal society seems to replicate much of that wished by Fromm:

> To seek enlightenment, intellectual or spiritual; to do good; to love and to be loved; to create and to teach; these are the highest purposes of humankind. If there is meaning in life, it lies here.
>
> (Monbiot, 2017, p.48)

But whatever the route is taken to advance the signs of sanity and thereby mental well-being, I contend that academics and clinicians and other readers of this book have a social and professional responsibility to try to make it happen.

References

Alvarez L, Alvarez W, Asaro F and Michel H (1980). Extraterrestrial Cause for the Cretaceous-Tertiary Extinction. *Science*, 208(4448), pp.1095–1108.

Clegg B (2017) *Big Data: How the Information Revolution is Transforming Our Lives*. London: Icon.

Frey D, MacNaughton G, Kaur A and Taborda E (2021) Crises as Catalyst: A New Social Contract Grounded in Worker Rights. *Health and Human Rights Journal*, 23(2), pp.153–165.

Fromm E (1955) *Sane Society*. New York: Rinehart.

Goldin I (2021) *Rescue: From Global Crisis to a Better World*. London: Spectre.

Lowery C and Fraass A (2019) Morphospace Expansion Paces Taxonomic Diversification After End Cretaceous Mass Extinction. *Nature Ecology and Evolution*, 3(6), pp.900–904.

Monbiot G (2017) *How Did We Get Into This Mess?: Politics, Equality, Nature*. London: Verso.

Morrall P (2020) *Insane Society: A Sociology of Mental Health*. Abingdon, UK: Routledge.

Saplakoglu Y (2019) Humans Will Never Live on an Exoplanet, Nobel Laureate Says. Here's Why. Live Science, 14th October. https://www.livescience.com/will-we-ever-live-exoplanet.html [accessed 8th January, 2022]

Snowden F (2020) (edition with Covid-19 preface) *Epidemics and Society: From the Black Death to the Present*. New Haven, CT, USA: Yale University Press.

Syed M (2019) *Rebel Ideas: The Power of Diverse Thinking*. London: John Murray.

Wilde L (2013) *Global Solidarity*. Edinburgh, UK: Edinburgh University Press.

Williams G (2011) *Angel of Death. The Story of Smallpox*. Basingstoke, UK: Palgrave Macmillan.

Yudkowsky E (2023) Pausing AI Developments Isn't Enough. We Need to Shut It All Down. *Time Magazine*, 29th March. https://time.com/6266923/ai-eliezer-yudkowsky-open-letter-not-enough/ [accessed 19th May, 2023]

Index

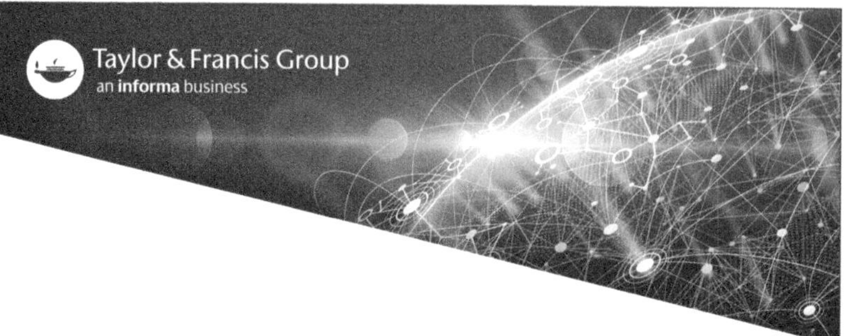

Taylor & Francis eBooks

www.taylorfrancis.com

A single destination for eBooks from Taylor & Francis
with increased functionality and an improved user
experience to meet the needs of our customers.

90,000+ eBooks of award-winning academic content in
Humanities, Social Science, Science, Technology, Engineering,
and Medical written by a global network of editors and authors.

TAYLOR & FRANCIS EBOOKS OFFERS:

A streamlined
experience for
our library
customers

A single point
of discovery
for all of our
eBook content

Improved
search and
discovery of
content at both
book and
chapter level

REQUEST A FREE TRIAL
support@taylorfrancis.com

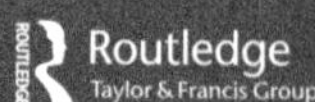

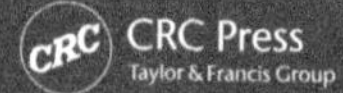

For Product Safety Concerns and Information please contact our
EU representative GPSR@taylorandfrancis.com Taylor & Francis
Verlag GmbH, Kaufingerstraße 24, 80331 München, Germany